Study toxicology through questions

John A. Timbrell
Glaxo Professor of Toxicology
School of Pharmacy
University of London

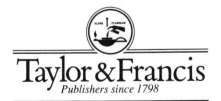

Taylor & Francis
Publishers since 1798

UK   Taylor & Francis Ltd., 1 Gunpowder Square, London EC4A 3DE

USA   Taylor & Francis Inc., 1900 Frost Road, Suite 101, Bristol, PA 19007

British Library Cataloguing in Publication Data

A catalogue record for this book is available from the British Library.

ISBN 0-7484-0695-6

Library of Congress Cataloguing Publication Data are available

Cover design by Amanda Barragry

Printed in Great Britain by T.J. International Ltd, Padstow

Contents

Preface   1

Introduction   3

1 **General toxicology**   5

          Multiple choice questions   5
          Short answer questions   6
   Answers   8
          Multiple choice   8
          Short answers   8

2 **Absorption, distribution and excretion of compounds**   13

          Multiple choice questions   13
          Short answer questions   17
          Problem solving questions   18
   Answers   22
          Multiple choice   22
          Short answers   24
          Problem solving   32

3 **Metabolism of compounds**   43

Contents

Multiple choice questions   43
Short answer questions   45
Problem solving questions   45
Answers   49
Multiple choice   49
Short answers   50
Problem solving   53

4 Factors affecting the toxicity of compounds 65

Multiple choice questions   65
Short answer questions   66
Problem solving questions   67
Answers   70
Multiple choice   70
Short answers   71
Problem solving   74

5 Toxic responses 83

Multiple choice questions   83
Short answer questions   87
Problem solving questions   88
Answers   90
Multiple choice   90
Short answers   92
Problem solving   94

6 Mechanisms of toxicity 99

Multiple choice questions   99
Problem solving questions   101
Answers   103
Multiple choice   103
Problem solving   104

7 Overall integration of the subject 111

Problem solving questions   111
Answers   120
Problem solving   120

Preface

This book has arisen from my involvement in teaching a BSc course in Toxicology and Pharmacology over the last 16 years. After devising questions of various types over this time I discovered how difficult and time consuming this can be. To refine the questions and put them together into a book with suggested answers seemed a useful endpoint which could be used by toxicologists at all levels.

I wish to thank Andy Shaw for his pharmacokinetics questions and Elaine Stott at Taylor & Francis for her help. However, I am especially grateful to Cathy Waterfield for producing all the figures and setting up the manuscript as camera ready copy, as well as for her patience.

London, April 1997.

Introduction

This book is intended for several types of audience:

- The student who needs a study aid for toxicology but wants more than a textbook as they need a self-testing regime.

- The teacher of toxicology who needs inspiration when composing questions for their students.

- The established toxicologist who wants to test their own knowledge or understanding.

It can be used at universities and colleges but also in industry for in-house training courses in toxicology which I know exist in some pharmaceutical and chemical companies.

The questions are a mixture of multiple choice, short answer and problem solving questions and are not meant to reflect a particular level of knowledge or development. Consequently some of the answers may be short whereas others are quite lengthy, even in the same question.

Although based loosely on *Principles of Biochemical Toxicology*, this book can be used alongside a number of standard toxicology texts which are listed below.

Suggested reading

Aldridge, W.N. (1996) *Mechanisms and Concepts in Toxicology*, London: Taylor & Francis.

Anderson, D. and Conning, D. (1996) *Experimental Toxicology. The Basic Principles*, 2nd edition, Cambridge: Royal Society of Chemistry.

Ballantyne, B., Marrs, T. and Turner, P. (eds) (1993) *General and Applied Toxicology*, Basingstoke: Macmillan.

Klaassen, C.D. (ed) (1996) *Cassarett and Doull's Toxicology*, 5th edition, New York: McGraw Hill.

Hayes, A.W. (ed) (1994) *Principles and Methods of Toxicology*, 3rd edition, London: Taylor & Francis.

Hodgson, E. and Levi, P.E. (eds) (1994) *Introduction to Biochemical Toxicology*, 2nd edition, Norwalk, Connecticut: Appleton & Lange.

Lu, F.C. (1996) *Basic Toxicology*, 3rd edition, London: Taylor & Francis.

Niesink, R.J.M., de Vries, J. and Hollinger, M.A. (eds) (1996) *Toxicology. Principles and Applications,* Boca Raton, U.S.A.: CRC Press.

Timbrell, J.A. (1991) *Principles of Biochemical Toxicology*, 2nd edition, London: Taylor & Francis.

1

General toxicology

MULTIPLE CHOICE QUESTIONS

Choose one answer which you think is the most appropriate.

Q1. A particular dose of a chemical A is toxic to animals *in vivo*. Another chemical B is not toxic when given at doses several orders of magnitude higher but when the two are given together the toxic response is greater than that of the given dose of A alone.

Is this an example of:

(a) antagonism
(b) synergism
(c) additivity
(d) potentiation
(e) none of the above

Q2. Which information may be gained from an acute toxicity study:

(a) the No Effect Level
(b) the LD_{50}
(c) the therapeutic index
(d) the target organ
(e) all of the above

Q3. The therapeutic index is usually defined as:

(a) TD_{50}/LD_{50}
(b) ED_{50}/LD_{50}
(c) LD_{50}/ED_{50}
(d) ED_{50}/TD_{50}
(e) LD_1/ED_{99}

Q4. 1000 p.p.m. is equivalent to 1%.

(a) True
(b) False

SHORT ANSWER QUESTIONS

Q5. The following is a list of antidotes. Match them up with the right poison.

Poison	Antidote/antagonist
Arsenic	Atropine/pralidoxime
Cyanide	Fuller's earth
Methanol	Dimercaprol
Paraquat	Ethanol
Parathion	Sodium nitrite/sodium thiosulphate
Lead	N-Acetylcysteine
Paracetamol	EDTA

Q6. Explain the following:

(a) LD_{50}
(b) dosage-response relationship
(c) therapeutic index
(d) NOEL

Q7. Explain using examples:

(a) synergism
(b) potentiation
(c) antagonism

Q8. Define the terms:

(a) TLV
(b) TD_{50}
(c) p.p.m.

Q9. Write notes on the following:

(a) ED_{50}
(b) ADI
(c) margin of safety

Q10. Define the terms *bioaccumulation* and *biomagnification* and state their importance in toxicology. Using one or more suitable examples, describe the properties that chemicals must possess if they are going to bioaccumulate.

ANSWERS

MULTIPLE CHOICE

A1. (d) Potentiation.

The compound B is not toxic yet when combined with A the toxicity is increased. Thus compound B potentiates the toxicity of A. This is distinct from synergism where both compounds are toxic but the toxicity of the combination is more than the sum.

A2. (e) All of the above.

A properly designed and carefully executed and observed acute toxicity study may give information on all of these parameters. The LD_{50} is now rarely required as an end in itself except for specific situations such as the design of pesticides. However, with a novel compound where the toxicity and lethality are unknown lethal doses may be administered to animals in preliminary toxicity studies. Consequently an LD_{50} could be calculated from such data.

A3. (c) LD_{50}/ED_{50}.

Therefore the bigger the therapeutic index the safer the drug. A better and more discriminating definition would be TD_{50}/ED_{50} in which the toxicity rather than the lethality is used for the numerator.

A4. (b) False. 1000 p.p.m. is 0.1%. Thus $\dfrac{1 \times 10^3}{1 \times 10^6} \times 100$.

SHORT ANSWERS

A5.

Poison	Antidote/antagonist
Arsenic	Dimercaprol
Cyanide	Sodium nitrite/sodium thiosulphate
Methanol	Ethanol
Paraquat	Fuller's earth
Parathion	Atropine/pralidoxime
Lead	EDTA
Paracetamol	N-Acetylcysteine

A6. (a) LD_{50} is the dose of a compound which is lethal for 50% of the population exposed to that compound. The value is determined from the dosage-response relationship by interpolation (see figure below).

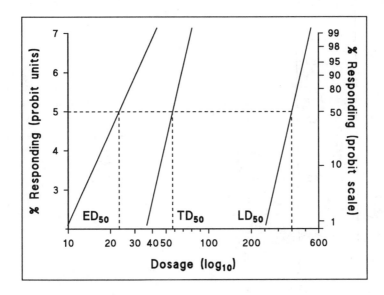

Figure: Answer 6 (a) and 6 (c). Dosage-response curves for pharmacological effect, toxic effect and lethal effect, illustrating the ED_{50}, TD_{50} and LD_{50}. The proximity of the curves for efficacy and toxicity indicates the margin of safety for the compound and the likelihood of toxicity occurring in certain individuals after doses necessary for the desired effect.

(b) Dosage (dose)-response relationship is the mathematical relationship between the dosage (dose) of a compound and the particular response measured. The response may be quantal (e.g. "all-or-none" such as lethality) or graded (e.g. inhibition of an enzyme). The relationship is typically a sigmoid curve. This reflects the fact that there are doses which have no effect and those which have a maximal effect (see figure page 10).

(c) Therapeutic index is an index of relative toxicity for a drug. Calculated as the LD_{50} or TD_{50} divided by the ED_{50}. Thus the greater the number, the less toxic the drug is relative to the pharmacologically effective dose (see figure above).

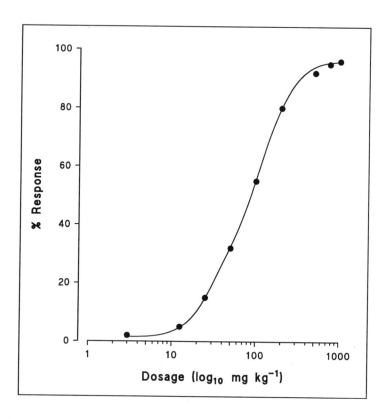

Figure: Answer 6 (b). Dosage-response curve.

(d) NOEL (the **N**o **O**bserved **E**ffect **L**evel) is the dose or exposure level of a chemical which has no demonstrable effect on a biological system. (NOAEL: No Observed Adverse Effect Level). The value may be derived from the dosageresponse relationship.

A7. (a) Synergism is the situation where the toxic effect of a mixture of two similarly toxic compounds is greater than the sum of the toxic effects of each component. For example, ethanol and carbon tetrachloride are both separately toxic to the liver. In combination the toxicity is greater than the sum of the individual toxicities.

(b) Potentiation is the situation where the toxic effect of a compound is greater when it is combined with another compound which is either non-toxic or differently toxic. For example, enzyme inducers such as phenobarbital increase paracetamol toxicity. Another example is the drug disulphiram which increases the toxicity of alcohol by blocking its metabolism and allowing an accumulation of acetaldehyde.

(c) Antagonism is the situation where one compound decreases the toxicity of another. Thus the overall effect of two compounds is less than additive. For example, the compound pyrazole decreases the toxicity of methanol in monkeys.

A8. (a) TLV: threshold limit value.

(b) TD_{50}: toxic dose for 50% of the exposed population.

(c) p.p.m.: parts per million. A unit of concentration in which there is a factor of 1 in 10^6, e.g. 1 μg g^{-1} or 1 mg kg^{-1}.

A9. (a) The ED_{50} is the dose of a compound which causes an effect in 50% of the organisms or a 50% response. This is usually a pharmacological, as distinguished from a toxicological, effect. The ED_{50} may be determined in a population of organisms or in an *in vitro* system. It may be a quantal ("all-or-none") response such as presence or absence of a pharmacological change or a graded response observed in the effect (see figure page 9).

(b) The ADI is defined as the "acceptable daily intake". This is usually applied to food additives or contaminants (such as pesticides). It is the calculated amount of a substance to which humans can be permitted to be exposed safely. It is calculated from the No Observed Adverse Effect Level (NOAEL) thus:

$$ADI = \frac{NOAEL \text{ mg kg}^{-1} \text{ day}^{-1}}{100}$$

The value of 100 is the safety factor which is applied. This takes into account the possible differences in susceptibility between the species used to determine the NOAEL and humans. A higher safety factor may be applied in some cases.

(c) The margin of safety is similar to the therapeutic index but more critical. Thus it is an indication of the difference between the dose or concentration of a drug required for the desired pharmacological effect and the dose associated with a toxic effect. It is calculated as follows:

$$\text{margin of safety} = \frac{TD_1}{ED_{99}} \text{ or } \frac{LD_1}{ED_{99}}$$

where TD_1 and LD_1 are the doses which are toxic or lethal for 1% of the population exposed and the ED_{99} is the dose which is effective in 99% of the population.

The margin of safety is more critical than the therapeutic index because it takes into account possible overlap in the dose response curves for pharmacological and toxicological effects.

A10. Bioaccumulation is the accumulation of a chemical substance in a biological organism. This is usually a reflection of the lipophilicity of the compound.

Biomagnification is the process whereby the concentration of a chemical substance in the organisms in a food chain increases towards the top of the chain. Thus the predator at the top of the food chain will have the highest concentration of pollutant.

For a compound to bioaccumulate it should be lipid soluble rather than water soluble. For example, the pesticide DDT will bioaccumulate in organisms exposed to it as it dissolves in the fat in adipose tissue. Second, the compound should be resistant to metabolism and therefore poorly excreted so that it is eliminated slowly from the organism. For example, polybrominated biphenyl compounds, such as those which contaminated livestock and people in Michigan in 1973, are very resistant to metabolism, are eliminated extremely slowly and so have very long half-lives. Continued exposure to such compounds will therefore result in accumulation in fat tissue.

2

Absorption, distribution and excretion of compounds

MULTIPLE CHOICE QUESTIONS

Choose one answer which you think is the most appropriate.

Q1. Some chemicals may be eliminated from the body by zero order kinetics. Which of the following would you expect for such chemicals:

(a) the composition of the metabolites changes quantitatively and qualitatively with dose
(b) the area under the plasma concentration vs time curve (AUC) is proportional to dose
(c) the half-life is increased as the dose increases
(d) the plasma level plotted against time shows an exponential relationship
(e) none of the above.

Q2. The parameter "volume of distribution" (V_D) may be determined for a chemical *in vivo*. Is it:

(a) equal to the water solubility of the chemical
(b) sometimes larger than the total body volume
(c) equal to the volume of total body water
(d) smaller than the total body water if highly bound in tissues
(e) none of the above

Q3. If particles of 20 μm diameter are inhaled, where in the respiratory system are they most likely to be deposited:

(a) alveoli
(b) nose
(c) trachea
(d) pulmonary bronchi
(e) terminal bronchioles

Q4. In an experimental study a volatile compound is given to animals. After low doses the compound is eliminated from the body as a metabolite in the urine. After high doses the metabolism is saturated. If the compound is radioactively labelled would you expect after a high dose:

(a) a decrease in radioactivity in the expired air
(b) an increase in radioactivity in the urine
(c) an increase in radioactivity in the faeces
(d) an increase in both urinary and expired radioactivity
(e) a shift in the proportion of radioactivity in urine to expired air

Q5. The half-life of a drug in the blood is determined by:

(a) the metabolism of the compound
(b) the volume of distribution
(c) plasma protein binding
(d) absorption of the drug
(e) urinary pH
(f) the total body clearance

Q6. The absorption of which of the following is facilitated by the prevailing pH in the stomach:

(a) weak organic bases
(b) strong acids
(c) weak organic acids
(d) strong bases
(e) none of the above

Q7. If the apparent volume of distribution of a drug in the body is greater than the total body water this is because:

(a) the drug is totally bound to plasma proteins
(b) the drug is very rapidly excreted
(c) the drug is bound to tissue components
(d) the drug is metabolised very quickly
(e) there is an error in one of the measurements

Q8. Which of the following does not contribute to the tissue distribution of a drug given orally:

(a) lipid solubility
(b) hepatic metabolism
(c) tissue blood flow
(d) plasma pH
(e) plasma protein binding

Q9. The phenomenon of enterohepatic recirculation of a chemical causes:

(a) a decrease in the volume of distribution
(b) an increase in the whole body half-life of the chemical
(c) a decrease in the metabolism of the compound
(d) a decrease in the whole body half-life
(e) zero order elimination of the chemical

Q10. The term "first-pass effect" means which of the following:

(a) the drug is excreted unchanged
(b) the drug is mostly metabolised by the gastrointestinal tract and/or liver before reaching the systemic circulation
(c) the drug is completely absorbed from the gastrointestinal tract
(d) the drug is excreted completely and very quickly by the kidneys
(e) none of the above

Q11. The oil/water partition coefficient of a chemical is an indication of:

(a) carcinogenicity
(b) long half-life
(c) potential to bioaccumulate
(d) low apparent volume of distribution
(e) chronic toxicity

Questions 12 and 13. Answer (a) if the statement is true and (b) if the statement is false.

Q12. The absorption of drugs into biological systems by passive diffusion is facilitated by ionisation of the compound.

Q13. Binding of drugs to proteins in the blood involves the formation of covalent bonds.

Questions 14 and 15. Select A if 1, 2 and 3 are correct
Select B if 1 and 3 are correct
Select C if 2 and 4 are correct
Select D if only 4 is correct
Select E if all four are correct

Q14. Which features of a chemical will favour accumulation in biological systems:

(1) binding to plasma proteins
(2) lipophilicity
(3) limited volume of distribution
(4) resistance to metabolism

Q15. When considering the chronic toxicity (but not acute toxicity) of a chemical which of the following must be considered:

(1) nature of the chemical
(2) half-life in the body
(3) dose of the chemical
(4) frequency of dosing

SHORT ANSWER QUESTIONS

Q16. Write notes on three of the following:

(a) volume of distribution
(b) binding of drugs to plasma proteins
(c) first-pass effect
(d) Fick's law of diffusion

Q17. Write notes on three of the following:

(a) the pH partition theory
(b) plasma half-life
(c) plasma clearance
(d) enterohepatic recirculation

Q18. Write notes on three of the following:

(a) total body burden
(b) area under the curve
(c) biliary excretion
(d) partition coefficient

Q19. Write notes on three of the following:

(a) carrier mediated transport
(b) inhibition of the drug metabolising enzymes
(c) glutathione
(d) the toxicology of DDT

Q20. Write notes on the toxicological importance of three of the following:

(a) blood flow to an organ
(b) bioavailability
(c) biomagnification
(d) gut bacteria

PROBLEM SOLVING QUESTIONS

Q21. The compound shown below is a potential new drug which is intended for oral administration. From the information given would you expect the compound to be well absorbed when given by the preferred route?

Would any metabolism take place and if so would this influence the absorption? Is the partition coefficient as determined useful information? Suggest further information about this compound which could be obtained and which would help in the prediction of extent of absorption.

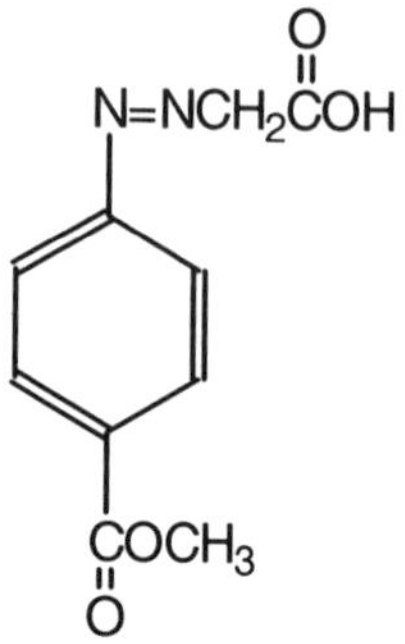

Figure: Question 21.

$pK_a = 2.1$; $\log P = 0.5$ (determined from the partition between chloroform and buffer pH 7.4).

Show **all** your calculations.

Q22. A 250 g rat was administered a compound (X) by intravenous infusion for two hours at a constant rate of 120 μg min^{-1}. Plasma concentrations (C_p) of X were monitored during the infusion and yielded the results given in the table below (page 19).

Determine the plasma half-life ($t_{1/2}$), the elimination rate constant (k_{el}) and the plasma clearance (Cl_p) of X.

When the infusion rate of X was increased, the calculated plasma clearance decreased. Interpret this finding and its possible toxicological significance.

Time from start of infusion (min)	C_P ($\mu g\ ml^{-1}$)
5	28
10	47
15	58
20	66
30	74
45	78
60	80
90	79
120	80

Q23. Therapeutic doses of antacids and phosphate binders taken orally contain high levels of aluminium which may have toxic consequences, particularly in patients with impaired renal function. In order to begin to assess this risk, Wilhelm and colleagues studied the toxicokinetics of aluminium (*Archives of Toxicology* (1992) **66**: 700−705). Five male Wistar rats (350−400 g) were each administered oral doses of aluminium lactate (volume = 0.7 ml; dose of aluminium = 12 mg kg^{-1}). Serial blood samples (100 μl) were drawn from a catheter in the right jugular vein at ten time points post-administration. The concentration of aluminium was determined in these samples by atomic absorption spectrometry. The following results were obtained:

Time after dosing (min)	Blood concentration of aluminium, C_B ($\mu g\ L^{-1}$)
20	18.0
40	28.0
60	33.0
80	34.0
100	33.0
200	23.0
300	11.0
400	5.7
500	2.9
600	1.4

A similar experiment was conducted where five rats were administered aluminium lactate by an intravenous bolus injection (dose of aluminium = 12 mg kg^{-1}). The area under the blood concentration of aluminium versus time graph (AUC) was calculated to be 709 mg h^{-1} L^{-1}. Using this information, determine the systemic bioavailability of aluminium after oral administration.

Q24. Human exposure to nicotine can occur from tobacco products, pharmaceuticals, e.g. nicotine chewing gum, nicotine-based insecticides, and dietary sources. Understanding the uptake and disposition of nicotine in humans is a vital step in assessing the potential adverse health effects of this chemical. To this end, the following experiment was performed. Six male Sprague-Dawley rats (mean weight = 271 g) were cannulated in the right jugular vein. Each rat was administered an intra-arterial injection of sterile saline containing 0.1 mg kg^{-1} nicotine. After dosing, each rat was housed in a metabolism cage and was allowed free access to food and water. Urine was collected for 12 h post-administration. Venous blood samples (250 µl) were drawn from the jugular vein at several time points after injection of nicotine. The blood samples were centrifuged at 10,500 g for 5 min and the plasma was removed. The concentration of nicotine in the plasma (see table below) and urine samples was determined by HPLC.

Time after dosing (min)	Mean plasma concentration of nicotine, C_P (ng ml^{-1})
2.5	41.5
5	33.5
10	26.8
15	23.5
20	21.0
30	18.5
60	12.5
120	5.8
180	2.7

Determine the following pharmacokinetic parameters for nicotine and briefly comment on its distribution:

(a) plasma half-life (h)
(b) volume of distribution (L kg^{-1} body weight)
(c) area under the curve (ng h^{-1} ml^{-1})
(d) plasma clearance (L h^{-1} kg^{-1} body weight)

Nicotine is eliminated by renal excretion and metabolism. If an average total of

2.3 µg nicotine was recovered from each rat's urine, determine values for the renal (Cl_{renal}) and metabolic $(Cl_{metabolic})$ clearance of nicotine.

Q25. The following data is for a new chemical intended as a pesticide for spraying onto crops. Determine the likelihood of the compound being absorbed by humans and discuss this data in relation to the possible routes of exposure.

The compound is a carboxylic acid derivative. It is a liquid which is miscible with water. It has a pK_a value of 5, a partition coefficient of log P, chloroform/water of 4 and its boiling point is 40°C.

ANSWERS

MULTIPLE CHOICE

A1. (c) The half-life is increased as the dose increases.

When a drug is eliminated by zero order kinetics this means that a constant amount is excreted per unit time. Therefore a graph of plasma level of drug against time is a straight line. In contrast to this for a drug eliminated by first order kinetics the equivalent graph would be an exponential curve (unless the plasma concentration is plotted on a log scale, in which case it becomes a straight line).

Because the amount excreted is constant for zero order kinetics, increasing the dose will increase the time taken for the plasma level to decrease by half, i.e. the half-life will increase.

A2. (b) Sometimes larger than the total body volume.

When a drug is bound to tissue components or sequestered in a tissue such as adipose tissue, the plasma level may be very low. Therefore the calculation of volume of distribution (V_D = dose/plasma level) yields a value which may be higher than the total body water. The volume of distribution may be equal to the total body water but this is not always the case.

A3. (d) Pulmonary bronchi.

Although particles of this size will be deposited in various parts of the respiratory system, it has been shown that the pulmonary bronchi will retain the greatest proportion.

A4. (e) A shift in the proportion of radioactivity in urine to expired air.

As the metabolism is saturated the proportion which can be excreted in the urine as water soluble metabolites will decline and therefore the proportion of the dose expired will increase. Although the amount of radioactivity excreted in the urine and expired will increase after a high dose, the proportions will not remain the same.

A5. (f) The total body clearance.

Although some of the other factors may have an effect on half-life, by definition the total body clearance is the major determining factor as this includes metabolism and excretion.

A6. (c) Weak organic acids.

In the stomach the pH is around 2 and at this pH weak acids will be non-ionised. Therefore passive absorption of the non-ionised acid will occur in the stomach.

A7. (c) The drug is bound to tissue components.

When a drug is bound to tissue components or sequestered in a tissue such as adipose tissue the plasma level may be very low. Therefore the calculation of volume of distribution gives a value which may be higher than the total body water.

A8. (b) Hepatic metabolism.

Metabolism of a drug simply removes it and therefore reduces the concentration in the blood but does not affect the distribution of the parent drug. All of the other factors may, under certain circumstances, facilitate the distribution of the parent drug into tissues.

A9. (b) An increase in the whole body half-life of the chemical.

Enterohepatic recirculation involves the excretion of a drug or metabolites into the bile followed by reabsorption from the intestine. This may occur several times. Therefore the overall elimination of the drug from the body is decreased because of this recycling between liver and intestine. Hence the whole body half-life is increased.

A10. (b) The drug is mostly metabolised by the gastrointestinal tract and/or liver before reaching the systemic circulation.

The "first-pass effect" is where a drug is removed by metabolism in the organ(s)/tissues through which it passes during absorption and before reaching the systemic circulation. This is commonly the gastrointestinal tract and liver but could also be the lungs or skin.

A11. (c) Potential to bioaccumulate.

The larger the partition coefficient the greater is the lipophilicity and this correlates with the bioaccumulation of the compound in fat tissue.

A12. (b) False.

Non-ionised compounds are more readily absorbed by passive diffusion as they more readily pass through the lipid bilayer parts of biological membranes.

A13. (b) False.

The binding of drugs to plasma proteins only rarely involves covalent binding. Usually ionic, hydrogen, hydrophobic or van der Waals' forces are involved.

A14. C.

Both lipophilicity and resistance to metabolism will favour accumulation of chemicals in biological systems. The former will result in sequestration in adipose tissue, the latter will decrease removal of the chemical by metabolism to polar, hydrophilic metabolites and loss by excretion.

A15. C.

Chemicals with a long half-life are more likely to accumulate on repeated dosing especially if the dosing interval is shorter than the half-life.

SHORT ANSWERS

A16. (a) The volume of distribution (V_D) is the volume of body fluid in which a chemical is apparently distributed after administration to an animal. It is calculated from either the dose and plasma (blood) concentration at a single time point or from the dose, area under the curve (AUC) and elimination rate constant (k_{el}):

$$V_D = \frac{\text{dose (mg)}}{\text{plasma concentration (mg L}^{-1})}.$$

The units are therefore in litres.

$$V_D = \frac{\text{dose}_{\text{i.v.}}}{C_0}$$

where the dose is given intravenously and the plasma concentration is measured or calculated at time zero (C_0). If the compound is distributed into a one compartment system then this calculation is sufficient. If the distribution is more complex then the following more rigorous calculation is appropriate:

$$V_D = \frac{\text{dose}_{\text{i.v.}} \times k_{el}}{\text{AUC}_{0-\infty}}$$

The volume of distribution does not necessarily equal a compartment and so may have a value higher than the total body water (40 litres for a human). This occurs if the plasma level is low, as when a drug is sequestered such as in adipose tissue. V_D is therefore known as apparent volume of distribution. The volume of distribution should not be calculated after the drug is administered orally as there may be incomplete absorption and/or first-pass metabolism.

(b) Drugs normally bind to plasma proteins non-covalently and in one of four ways:
(i) by ionic bonds in which there is bonding between charged groups or atoms and opposite charges on the protein
(ii) by hydrogen bonds where a hydrogen atom attached to an electronegative atom (e.g. O) is shared with another electronegative atom
(iii) by hydrophobic interactions in which two non-polar, hydrophillic groups associate and mutually repel water
(iv) by van der Waals' forces; these are weak forces acting between the nucleus of one atom and the electrons of another.

There may be several molecules of drug bound to one protein molecule and strength may vary depending on the type of binding. However, binding is normally reversible. The protein commonly involved in binding is albumin. Binding to plasma proteins may increase the half-life and limit the distribution and metabolism of a drug. Drugs bound to plasma proteins may be displaced by other drugs, leading to a large rise in the free concentration in the plasma. Similarly increasing the dose of a drug which is bound extensively to plasma proteins may saturate the binding sites and lead to a sudden increase in plasma level.

(c) The first-pass effect is the extensive metabolism of a drug either by the organ of absorption or the liver following oral administration. This may lead to the situation where very little of the parent drug is distributed around the body. Thus after oral absorption a drug may be metabolised by the gastrointestinal tract and/or the liver before reaching the systemic circulation. Therefore if the parent drug is active, little may reach the target site. If the metabolism is saturable, however, increasing the dose may dramatically increase the systemic exposure. The lungs and skin, the other organs of absorption, may also carry out first-pass metabolism.

The figure below shows the effect of first-pass metabolism of a compound after oral and intravenous administration.

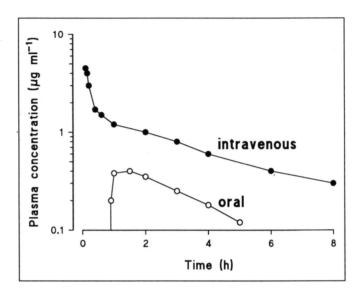

Figure: Answer 16 (c). Effect of first-pass metabolism.

(d) Fick's law of diffusion describes the relationship between the rate of diffusion of a chemical across a membrane and certain characteristics of the membrane. In the context of toxicology and drug disposition it relates to passage across a cell membrane by simple diffusion. Thus:

$$\text{rate of diffusion} = \frac{KA\,(C_2 - C_1)}{d}$$

where K is the diffusion coefficient, A is the surface area, C_2 is the concentration of compound outside the membrane, C_1 is the concentration of compound on the inside of the membrane and d is the thickness of the membrane. The diffusion coefficient will incorporate physicochemical characteristics of the chemical such as lipophilicity, size, shape, etc.

A17. (a) The pH partition theory states that only non-ionised lipid soluble compounds will be absorbed by passive diffusion down a concentration gradient. For absorption of a compound to occur through a biological membrane the compound must be lipid soluble and the concentration on the inside of the membrane should be lower than on the outside. Compounds which are ionised at the pH of the biological environment will not normally be able to pass through the membrane by passive diffusion although they may be substrates for active transport processes.

(b) Plasma half-life ($t_{1/2}$) is the time taken for the concentration of a drug in the plasma (blood) to decrease by half from a given point. It reflects the rates at which the various *in vivo* dynamic processes of distribution, metabolism and excretion are taking place. It can be determined from a plot of the plasma level against time by measurement (see figure below) or from the equation:

$$\text{half-life} = \frac{0.693}{k_{el}}$$

where k_{el} is determined from the slope of the graph log plasma concentration vs time (slope $= -k_{el}/2.303$).

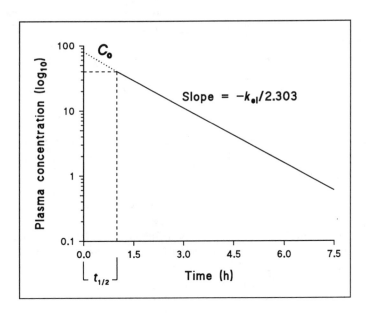

Figure: Answer 17 (b). Log_{10} plasma concentration time profile for a foreign compound after intravenous administration. The plasma half-life ($t_{1/2}$) and the elimination rate constant (k_{el}) of the compound can be determined from the graph as shown.

The half-life is an important measurement as changes in this parameter may reflect, for example, saturation of metabolism or excretion. A knowledge of the half-life is also important in relation to repeat dosing with a drug. If the dosing interval is shorter than the half-life then accumulation will occur.

(c) Plasma clearance is a derived parameter and is an indication of the rate of removal of a drug from the blood or other body fluid by excretion or metabolism. It is calculated from the area under the plasma concentration vs time curve (AUC):

$$\text{clearance} = \frac{\text{dose}}{\text{AUC}}$$

Therefore, the units are volume/unit time, e.g. ml min^{-1}. Thus a plasma clearance of 100 ml min^{-1} means that 100 ml of plasma is completely cleared of the drug every minute. Therefore the higher the clearance, the more efficiently and rapidly a chemical is removed from the fluid.

(d) The term enterohepatic recirculation describes the process whereby a chemical in the body is secreted from the liver into the bile, passes into the small intestine and is then reabsorbed into the blood stream. For example, the chemical may be secreted into bile as a polar conjugate following metabolism in the liver. Then when the bile enters the intestine this conjugate is cleaved by bacterial metabolism and the original drug or other fragment is reabsorbed from the intestine and re-enters the liver via the portal circulation. This process may be repeated several times and therefore it prolongs the exposure of the liver and rest of the body to the compound. If the compound has been administered orally, very little may reach the systemic circulation. The plasma level profile may reflect the process by showing peaks at various times, corresponding to reabsorption, rather than a smooth decline.

A18. (a) The total body burden of a chemical is the amount remaining in the body at any one time. It can be calculated from the volume of distribution and the plasma concentration at the time:

$$\text{total body burden (mg)} = \text{plasma concentration (mg L}^{-1}) \times V_D \text{ (L)}$$

(b) The area under the curve (AUC) for a chemical is determined from the graph of the plasma (blood) concentration plotted against time on normal rectilinear graph paper. It is the area enclosed by the plasma level line and the x or the x and y axes (see figure page 29). It can be determined by computer or by dividing the area into trapezoids and calculating the area of each (e.g. $C_0 - C_1 = C' \times t_1 - t_0$). The parameter AUC therefore gives an indication of overall exposure to the chemical over time.

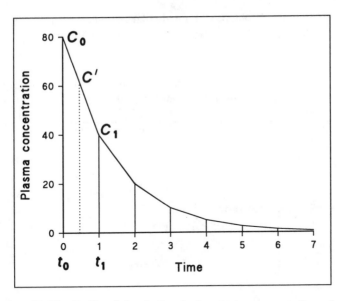

Figure: Answer 18 (b). Profile of the decline in the plasma concentration of a foreign compound with time after intravenous administration. The area under the curve (AUC) may be calculated by adding the individual areas of trapezoids.

(c) Biliary excretion is the elimination of chemicals from the body in the bile. The secretion of bile from the liver involves active transport of substances from the hepatocyte. Therefore the excretion of foreign chemicals may be saturated by high concentrations or affected by metabolic dysfunction in the liver. Excretion of chemicals into the bile is affected by the molecular weight of the chemical, its charge and the species of animal. Thus there is a molecular weight threshold which varies between species (approximately 300 in rats but more like 500 in humans). Anions, cations and neutral compounds are transported by different active transport systems. Some compounds may also be excreted by diffusion.

(d) The partition coefficient of a chemical is a measure of its lipid solubility. It is determined by measuring the amount of a chemical present in the aqueous and organic phases after an aqueous solution of the chemical is shaken with an organic solvent (or oil). The ratio of the concentration in the organic phase to the concentration in the aqueous phase is the partition coefficient. It may be expressed as the $\log_{10}$ of this ratio ($\log P$). The aqueous phase may be water or buffer at a particular pH (e.g. 7.4 for relevance to biological systems). The organic phase used is often chloroform although other organic solvents such as octanol and even olive oil may be used. Clearly the combination must be specified when the value is quoted.

A19. (a) Carrier mediated transport relates to the transport of foreign compounds (and endogenous compounds) across biological membranes. The process involves a carrier system which is specific for a particular chemical structure or similar types of structures. The other features are that the system requires energy in the form of ATP, it can operate against a concentration gradient, similar compounds will compete for transport and it can be inhibited by metabolic poisons such as cyanide. Finally, it may be saturated by increased concentrations. Therefore transport by this mechanism shows zero order kinetics (see figure below).

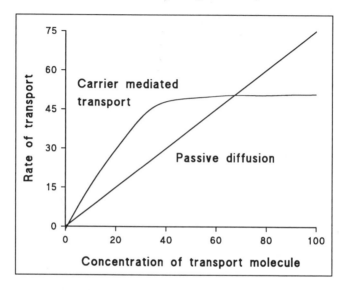

Figure: Answer 19 (a). Comparison of the kinetics of carrier mediated transport and passive diffusion.

(b) The drug metabolising enzymes are important in toxicology because they are often involved in detoxication of foreign and potentially toxic compounds. Therefore inhibition of these enzymes can result in increased exposure of the body to the chemical and prolonged half-life. This may lead to increased toxicity to the compound if the parent chemical is toxic. However, if a metabolite is toxic then inhibition of these enzymes may lead to decreased toxicity.

(c) Glutathione is a tripeptide found in most mammalian tissues, but especially the liver. Here it has a concentration of 5 mM or greater. The amino acids which constitute glutathione are glutamic acid, cysteine and glycine. The cysteine has a free SH (sulphydryl) group which is crucial to the function of glutathione. The molecule may exist in oxidised (GSH) or reduced (GSSG) form. In the latter case the SH group is oxidised and two glutathione molecules combine together. Glutathione is important in toxicology for a number of reasons: a) it is conjugated enzymatically with many chemicals which are then excreted into the bile unchanged or after metabolism into the urine as cysteine or *N*-acetylcysteine conjugates; b) it reacts with and detoxifies reactive chemical intermediates produced by metabolism

30

that are then excreted into the bile or, after metabolism as cysteine or
N-acetylcysteine conjugates, into the urine; c) it can act as an antioxidant and
reduce and thereby detoxify free radicals and similar reactive intermediates (such
as hydrogen peroxide), in the process becoming oxidised to oxidised GSH or
GSSG. In these ways it protects the cell against damage.

(d)   DDT is the insecticide dichloro-diphenyl-trichloroethane.   It is very
hydrophobic and hence very lipophilic (lipid soluble).   It is therefore persistent in
the environment and bioaccumulates in the food chain.   It is metabolised to other
chemicals which are more persistent, such as the metabolite DDE.   It is toxic to
insects by affecting the transport of ions in nerves but is relatively non-toxic to
birds, mammals and other organisms.   However, when it accumulates it becomes
toxic to birds and other organisms higher in the food chain.   It has been detected
in human breast milk where it may be concentrated and so babies may be exposed
to the substance at higher levels than adults.   Repeated exposure to DDT leads to
induction of the microsomal enzymes and this may be the cause of the thinning of
the shells of birds' eggs.   Thus increased/altered metabolism of steroid hormones
involved in egg production has been demonstrated.

A20. (a) The blood flow to an organ is an important factor in the exposure of that
organ to a chemical.   Thus the delivery of the chemical will depend on this and so
poorly perfused organs or tissues will have lower exposure to chemicals than highly
perfused organs.   Blood flow to an organ is also important toxicologically because
of clearance of the chemical by that organ.   Thus if a chemical is removed from the
blood by an organ such as the liver (metabolism) or the kidney (excretion), then the
blood flow is an important determinant of the clearance.   Indeed clearance by an
organ cannot be greater than the blood flow to that organ.

(b) The bioavailability of a chemical is the proportion of the dose of the drug or
other chemical which reaches the systemic circulation and is therefore available to
the organism following absorption from a particular site.   It can be determined
experimentally by comparing the AUC after oral and after intravenous dosing and
is often expressed as a percentage:

$$\frac{AUC_{oral} \times 100}{AUC_{i.v.}}$$

Thus a chemical which is well absorbed from the gastrointestinal tract would have
a bioavailability of perhaps 90%.   Bioavailability is an important concept in
toxicology as it is not the administered dose which is of prime importance but the
amount of chemical to which the organism is exposed.

(c)   Biomagnification is the term describing the phenomenon of increasing concentration of a lipophilic chemical in the organisms of an ecosystem. Thus the concentration of the chemical increases as the complexity of the organism increases. For example, the concentration of DDT in a predatory bird such as hawk may be many times higher than in fish which may be again many fold higher than in plankton.   This phenomenon results from the accumulation of the lipophilic chemical in the fat of organisms exposed. When these organisms are eaten by other, larger organisms, the chemical accumulates in the fat of these organisms also.

(d)   The gut bacteria are important toxicologically because of their ability to metabolise chemicals. This may be important when a chemical is administered orally and the bacteria of the gastrointestinal tract convert the compound into metabolites that may be toxic or that may have different absorption characteristics. Alternatively the gut bacteria may be important in metabolising compounds secreted into the bile and eliminated into the gastrointestinal tract.   This may result in cleavage of conjugates such as glucuronides and reabsorption of the original compound (aglycone).

PROBLEM SOLVING

A21. The compound shown is an acid and therefore potentially would be absorbed in the stomach in humans where the pH is about 2. The pK_a is 2.1. Therefore the drug will be approximately 50% non-ionised in the stomach. However, the amount of drug ionised in the stomach and intestine can be calculated using the Henderson-Hasselbach equation as follows:

The drug is an acid therefore it will ionise as follows:

$$R\text{-COOH} = R\text{-COO}^- + H^+$$

For an acid:

$$pH = pK_a + \log \frac{[A^-]}{[AH]}$$

In the stomach pH = 2 and for the compound $pK_a = 2.1$.

$$2 = 2.1 + \log \frac{[A^-]}{[AH]}$$

Therefore:

$$-0.1 = \log \frac{[A^-]}{[AH]} \qquad \text{Antilog} -0.1 = \frac{[A^-]}{[AH]} = 0.79.$$

32

In other words the ratio of ionised to non-ionised drug is less than 1, meaning that more than half is in the non-ionised form. If $[A^-] = 1$, then $[AH] = 1.26$ and the drug is 55% non-ionised. Therefore provided the drug is reasonably lipid soluble it is likely to be absorbed in the stomach by passive diffusion because there will be a concentration gradient between the stomach and blood. In the intestine the pH is approximately 6, therefore the same calculation results in the ratio:

$$\frac{[A^-]}{[AH]} = 0.0001.$$

This means that the compound is almost completely ionised (99.99%) and therefore will not be absorbed by passive diffusion.

From the structure of the compound it would be predicted that metabolism would take place in the gastrointestinal tract, in particular in the intestine. This would be the result of action of the gut bacteria which would cleave the azo link as shown (see figure below). This would alter the characteristics of the drug, which would now become basic rather than acidic. Therefore it would be more likely to be absorbed in the intestine where the pH is about 6. Another possibility is that the ester group might be cleaved by the acid in the stomach or bacterial enzymes. This would yield a different compound which might be less lipid soluble, having another acid grouping, or, if also subject to azo bond cleavage, would acquire both acidic and basic groups and become a zwitterion. This probably would be less well absorbed.

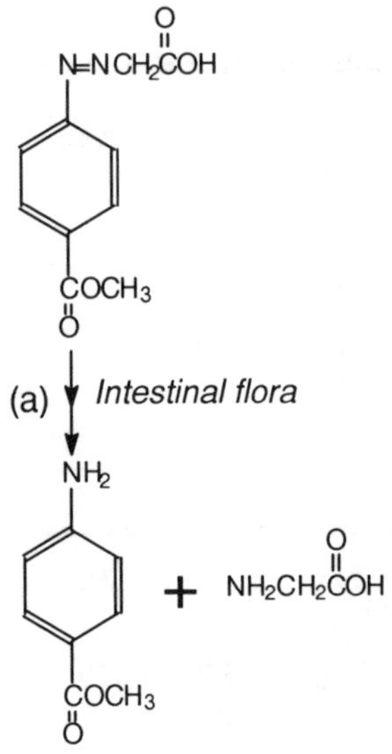

Figure: Answer 21. Metabolism by intestinal flora. (a) is azoreductase.

The value of log P, the log of the partition coefficient, is given as 0.5. This is defined as being determined between chloroform and buffer at pH 7.4. This means that the ratio of the concentration of drug in the organic phase (chloroform) to the concentration in the aqueous phase (buffer, pH 7.4) is 3.16 (antilog 0.5). Therefore more of the compound dissolves in the organic phase and so one can conclude that the drug has some lipid solubility. However, from the structure of the drug and its pK_a value it is clear that the compound will be ionised at pH 7.4. Therefore the partition coefficient will be higher if measured at an acidic pH such as 2 which is more relevant to the likely site of absorption (stomach) and at which ionisation will be suppressed.

From the information given, however, it is a reasonable conclusion that the drug will be absorbed from the stomach after an oral dose. Although the partition coefficient is useful, a better estimate of likely absorption would be possible with a partition coefficient measured in buffer at pH 2.

Other information which would be useful is a knowledge of the water solubility. If the compound is insoluble in water this will reduce the absorption from the stomach, which is an aqueous environment.

A22. Log C_P was plotted against infusion time (line A, see figure page 35). The steady state plasma concentration $(C_{SS}) = 80$ µg ml^{-1}.

Calculation of $t_{1/2}$

Time (min)	C_P (µg ml^{-1})	$C_{SS} - C_P$ (µg ml^{-1})
0	0[a]	80
5	28	52
10	47	33
15	58	22
20	66	14
30	74	6
45	78	2
60	80	0

[a] This assumes that no X is present in the blood before the infusion proceeds.

Log $(C_{SS} - C_P)$ was plotted against infusion time and displayed a linear relationship (line B, see figure page 35). From this graph, the $t_{1/2}$ of X was calculated to be **8 min**.

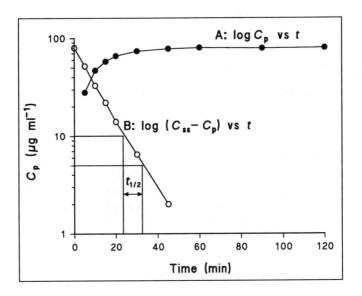

Figure: Answer 22. Graph to determine the half-life, elimination constant and plasma clearance of X.

Calculation of k_{el}

$$k_{el} = \frac{\ln 2}{t_{\frac{1}{2}}} = \frac{0.693}{8 \text{ min}} = 0.087 \text{ min}^{-1}.$$

Calculation of Cl_p

$$Cl_p = \frac{\text{rate of elimination}}{C_p}$$

When $C_p = C_{ss}$, rate of elimination = rate of infusion. Therefore,

$$Cl_p = \frac{\text{rate of infusion}}{C_{ss}} = \frac{120 \text{ µg min}^{-1}}{80 \text{ µg ml}^{-1}} = 1.5 \text{ ml min}^{-1}.$$

Interpretation

If the elimination of X is a passive process, e.g. glomerular filtration in the kidney, then raising the infusion rate of X will increase the plasma concentration of X, which will in turn cause a proportional rise in the rate of elimination of X. This is apparent from the equation:

$$\text{rate of elimination} = C_p \times Cl_p$$

where plasma clearance is a constant. A similar relationship would exist were X eliminated by an active process, e.g. renal secretion or metabolism, but where the process remained unsaturated.

However, if the elimination of X becomes saturated as the plasma concentration rises, then the rate of elimination will reach a maximum and will be constant. Consequently, increasing the infusion rate further will result in a decrease in plasma clearance (as reported here) and dramatic rises in the concentration of X in the blood and tissues, possibly with toxicological consequences. This is referred to as dose-dependent or non-linear kinetics and is an important concept in toxicology as it often coincides with the dose-response of toxic compounds, e.g. saccharin, cyclohexylamine and 2,4,5-trichlorophenoxyacetic acid.

A23. Log C_B was plotted against time after oral dosing (see graph below).

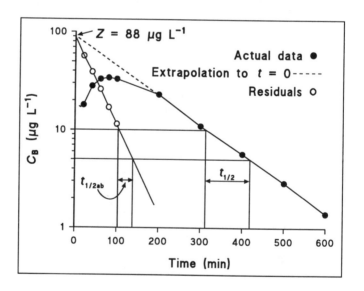

Figure: Answer 23. Graph used to calculate the biological half-life of aluminium.

The log-linear section of this graph was used as shown to calculate the plasma half-life of aluminium: $t_{\frac{1}{2}} = \mathbf{100}$ **min**.

From this the elimination rate constant can be calculated:

elimination rate constant (k_{el}) = $\dfrac{\ln 2}{t_{\frac{1}{2}}}$ = $\dfrac{0.693}{100\ \text{min}}$ = **0.0069 min⁻¹**.

The log-linear portion of the graph can be extrapolated to intersect the y axis at zero time. The value at the intercept (Z) is 88 µg L⁻¹.

In order to determine the bioavailability the AUC needs to be determined. For this the absorption rate constant has to be calculated. This can be determined using the method of residuals.

Method of residuals

Time (min)	C_B (µg ml⁻¹)	Extrapolated value (µg L⁻¹) from graph	Residuals: extrapolated value − C_B (µg L⁻¹)
20	18.0	75.0	57.0
40	28.0	67.0	39.0
60	33.0	59.0	26.0
80	34.0	51.0	17.0
100	33.0	44.5	11.5

The values in column 4 above (the residuals) were plotted against time and displayed a linear relationship (see graph page 36). From this graph, $t_{\frac{1}{2}ab}$ was calculated to be **35 min**. From this the absorption rate constant can be calculated:

absorption rate constant (k_{ab}) = $\dfrac{\ln 2}{t_{\frac{1}{2}ab}}$ = $\dfrac{0.693}{35\ \text{min}}$ = **0.0198 min⁻¹**.

Calculation of area under the curve (AUC_oral)

$$\text{AUC}_{oral} = \frac{Z}{k_{el}} - \frac{Z}{k_{ab}}$$

$$= \frac{88\ \text{µg L}^{-1}}{0.0069\ \text{min}^{-1}} - \frac{88\ \text{µg L}^{-1}}{0.0198\ \text{min}^{-1}}$$

$$= 8309\ \text{µg min}^{-1}\ \text{L}^{-1}$$

$$\text{AUC}_{oral} = \textbf{0.138 mg h}^{-1}\ \textbf{L}^{-1}.$$

Calculation of the systemic oral bioavailability of aluminium (F_{oral})

$$F_{oral} = \frac{AUC_{oral} \times dose_{iv}}{AUC_{iv} \times dose_{oral}}$$

Note AUC_{iv} is given as 709 mg h^{-1} L^{-1} therefore

$$F_{oral} = \frac{0.138 \text{ mg h}^{-1} \text{ L}^{-1} \times 12 \text{ mg kg}^{-1}}{709 \text{ mg h}^{-1} \text{ L}^{-1} \times 12 \text{ mg kg}^{-1}}$$

$$F_{oral} = \textbf{1.9 x 10}^{-4}$$

i.e. 0.019% of the oral dose reaches the general circulation.

A24. (a) Calculation of plasma half-life ($t_{\frac{1}{2}}$)

Log C_p was plotted against time after dosing (see graph below). The log-linear section of this graph was used as shown to calculate the plasma half-life of nicotine in SpragueDawley rats; $t_{\frac{1}{2}} = 54$ min = **0.9 h**.

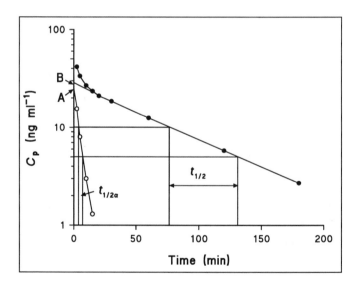

Figure: Answer 24. Graph to calculate the plasma half-life, volume of distribution and plasma clearance of nicotine.

(b) Calculation of volume of distribution (V_D)

The log-linear portion of the graph was extrapolated to zero time. The value at the intercept (B) was 27 ng ml^{-1}.

$$V_D = \frac{\text{dose}}{B} = \frac{0.1 \times 10^6 \text{ ng kg}^{-1}}{27 \text{ ng ml}^{-1}} = 3704 \text{ ml kg}^{-1} = \textbf{3.7 L kg}^{-1}.$$

(c) Calculation of area under the curve (AUC)

Hybrid elimination rate constant $\beta = \dfrac{\ln 2}{t_{\frac{1}{2}}} = \dfrac{0.693}{0.9 \text{ h}} = \textbf{0.77 h}^{-1}$.

Method of residuals

Time (min)	C_P (ng ml^{-1})	Extrapolated value (ng ml^{-1})	Residual: C_P − extrapolated value (ng ml^{-1})
2.5	41.5	26.0	15.5
5	33.5	25.5	8.0
10	26.8	23.8	3.0
15	23.5	22.2	1.3

The residuals were plotted against time and displayed a linear relationship (see graph page 38). The value at intercept A (zero time) = 25.5 ng ml^{-1}. From this graph $t_{\frac{1}{2}\alpha}$ was calculated to be 3.5 min (0.058 h).

Hybrid elimination rate constant $\alpha = \dfrac{\ln 2}{t_{\frac{1}{2}\alpha}} = \dfrac{0.693}{0.058 \text{ h}} = 11.95 \text{ h}^{-1}$.

$$\text{AUC} = \frac{A}{\alpha} + \frac{B}{\beta} = \frac{25.5 \text{ ng ml}^{-1}}{11.95 \text{ h}^{-1}} + \frac{27 \text{ ng ml}^{-1}}{0.77 \text{ h}^{-1}}$$

$$= \textbf{37.2 ng h}^{-1} \textbf{ ml}^{-1}.$$

(d) Calculation of plasma clearance (Cl_P)

$$Cl_P = \frac{\text{dose}}{\text{AUC}} = \frac{10^5 \text{ ng kg}^1}{37.2 \text{ ng h}^{-1} \text{ ml}^1} = 2688 \text{ ml h}^{-1} \text{ kg}^{-1}$$

$$= \textbf{2.69 L h}^{-1} \textbf{ kg}^{-1}.$$

Calculation of renal and metabolic clearance

Mean mass of nicotine recovered in each rat's urine $=$ 2.3 μg nicotine.

Mean mass of nicotine given to each rat = dose (μg kg^{-1}) x mean rat weight (kg/rat)

$\qquad$ = 0.1 x 10^3 μg kg^{-1} x 0.271 kg

$\qquad$ = 27.1 μg nicotine/rat.

Therefore, the fraction of the dose which is excreted in the urine

$\qquad$ = $\dfrac{2.3 \text{ μg}}{27.1 \text{ μg}}$ = 0.085 (i.e. 8.5%).

Cl_{renal} = Cl_{p} x the fraction of the dose which is renally excreted

$\qquad$ = 2.69 L h^{-1} kg^{-1} x 0.085 = **0.23 L h^{-1} kg^{-1}**.

Assuming that the remaining nicotine is cleared by metabolism, $Cl_{\text{metabolic}}$ will equal the difference between the plasma clearance and the renal clearance:

$Cl_{\text{p}} - Cl_{\text{renal}}$ = 2.69 L h^{-1} kg^{-1} − 0.23 l h^{-1} kg^{-1} = **2.46 L h^{-1} kg^{-1}**.

A25. As the compound is a pesticide for spraying it is likely to be a hazard by absorption through skin contact and/or inhalation.

The boiling point is 40°C which means that although it is a liquid at normal ambient temperature, it is volatile and so in hot countries it will be likely to exist mostly as a vapour.

The lipid solubility is high log P = 4, therefore the partition coefficient (chloroform:water) is 10,000 which means that the ratio of the proportion of compound distributed in chloroform to water is 10,000:1. Consequently it is likely that absorption via the lungs will be efficient. Skin absorption may also be efficient unless the compound is sequestered in subcutaneous fat due to the high lipid solubility.

However, as the compound is an acid with a pK_{a} of 5, it will be ionised in the blood.

Using the Henderson-Hasselbach equation:

$$pH = pK_a + \log \frac{A^-}{HA}$$

At pH 7.4 (blood):

$$7.4 = 5 + \log \frac{A^-}{HA}$$

Therefore:

$$7.4 - 5 = \log \frac{A^-}{HA} = 2.4$$

$$\frac{A^-}{HA} = \text{antilog } 2.4 = 251.$$

Therefore the ratio of ionised (A^-) to non-ionised (HA) compound is 251:1. Consequently there will be ionisation pressure facilitating the absorption from the lungs and skin because ionisation will maintain the concentration gradient.

Although exposure through the gastrointestinal tract is less likely absorption may occur in the stomach (pH 2) where the compound will be mostly non-ionised:

$$2 = 5 + \log \frac{A^-}{HA}$$

$$-3 = \log \frac{A^-}{HA}, \quad \text{antilog } -3 = \frac{A^-}{HA} = 0.001.$$

Therefore the compound is mainly (99.9%) non-ionised in the stomach and would be likely to be absorbed, especially as it will be ionised in the plasma, and so there will be a concentration gradient. In the intestine (pH 6) the compound would be approximately 90% ionised and so would be less likely to be absorbed.

Overall therefore this compound will present a significant hazard because it is likely to be absorbed from several sites.

3

Metabolism of compounds

MULTIPLE CHOICE QUESTIONS

Choose one answer which you think is the most appropriate.

Q1. If a chemical which is directly cytotoxic is detoxified by metabolism via the microsomal enzyme system and the activity of this system correlates with basal metabolic rate, which would you expect to be the species most sensitive to the chemical? All the species are given an equivalent dose on a weight basis.

(a) man
(b) mouse
(c) rat
(d) dog
(e) rabbit

Q2. Metabolism of a foreign chemical will lead to:

(a) accumulation of the chemical in the tissues
(b) increased excretion in urine
(c) decreased toxicity
(d) altered chemical structure
(e) increased toxicity

Q3. Cytochrome P450 is an enzyme which:

(a) is found in lysosomes
(b) is responsible for the conjugation of drugs

(c) is a central part of the drug metabolising system
(d) is one of the enzymes in the mitochondrial electron transport chain
(e) (c) and (d) are correct

Q4. Phase 2 metabolism usually involves:

(a) microsomal enzymes
(b) decreasing the polarity of a chemical
(c) increasing the toxicity of compounds
(d) the addition of an endogenous moiety
(e) hydrolysis

Q5. Glutathione is which of the following:

(a) a protein
(b) a tripeptide
(c) an enzyme involved in detoxication
(d) a substance found in the kidneys
(e) a vitamin

Q6. Answer (a) if the statement is true and (b) if the statement is false.

Cytochrome P450 mainly catalyses the phase 1 metabolism of chemicals.

Q7. The microsomal enzyme system is responsible for the metabolism of foreign compounds. Which of the following are essential aspects of this system?

Select A if 1, 2 and 3 are correct
Select B if 1 and 3 are correct
Select C if 2 and 4 are correct
Select D if only 4 is correct
Select E if all four are correct

(1) magnesium ions
(2) the addition of two electrons
(3) molecular oxygen
(4) the substrate is bound to an iron atom in the active site

SHORT ANSWER QUESTIONS

Q8. Write notes on three of the following:

(a) cytochrome P450
(b) glutathione
(c) phase 3 metabolism
(d) the NIH shift

Q9. Write short notes on three of the following:

(a) enzyme mediated dealkylation
(b) alcohol dehydrogenase
(c) glucuronic acid conjugation
(d) phase 1 and 2 metabolism

Q10. Write notes on three of the following:

(a) *N*-acetyltransferase
(b) epoxide hydrolase
(c) glutathione-*S*-transferase
(d) taurine

PROBLEM SOLVING QUESTIONS

Q11. The structure shown below is a hypothetical new drug designed for oral administration. Show diagrammatically the routes of metabolism you would predict. Name the enzymes which catalyse any pathways you show.

$$CH_2OCH_2CH_2OH$$

Figure: Question 11.

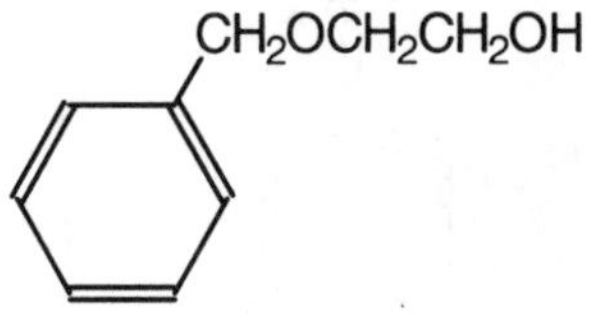

Q12. Discuss the phase 1 and phase 2 metabolic pathways which the foreign compound shown below might be expected to undergo in a mammalian organism. Indicate both the expected metabolites and the enzymes involved.

Figure: Question 12.

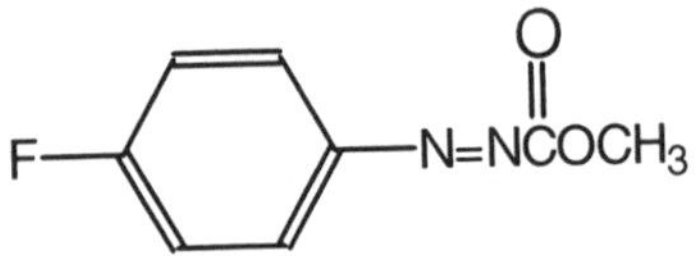

Q13. The compound shown below is a potential new drug for veterinary use in various animals. Show diagrammatically the possible routes of metabolism for this compound and the enzymes responsible. The route of administration for this compound has not yet been decided. Which route would you advise the pharmaceutical scientists to choose and why?

Figure: Question 13.

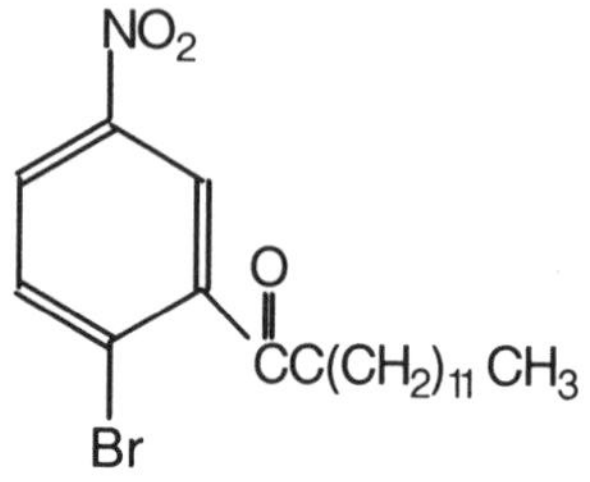

Q14. The compound shown below is a new chemical entity produced by a drug company. Show the routes of metabolism you would predict for this compound and indicate what enzymes catalyse the reactions. The route of administration for this compound has not yet been decided but may be oral or by skin application. Would there be any difference in the metabolism of this compound by the two routes of administration? Would any of the metabolites you have predicted be likely to be toxic? Explain your answers.

Figure: Question 14.

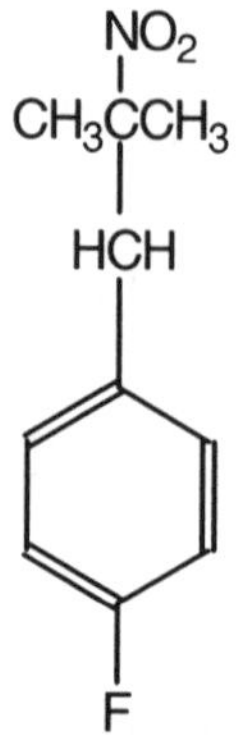

Q15. The compound shown below is a potential new drug. You have been asked to predict the metabolites. Show this diagrammatically and indicate the enzymes involved. Are any of the metabolites likely to be toxic?

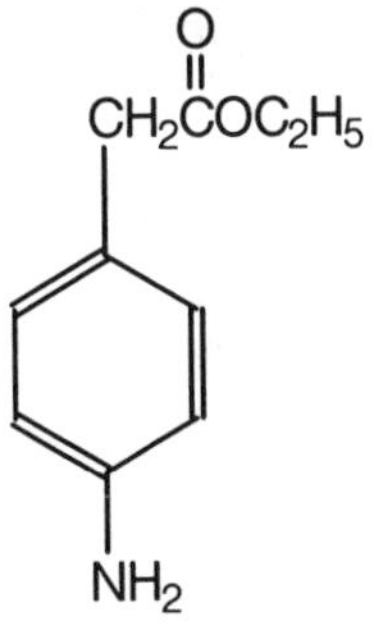

$$CH_2COC_2H_5$$

Figure: Question 15.

NH_2

Q16. The structure shown below is a potential rodenticide. Rodent pests will eat the compound in food. Suggest ways in which the compound might be metabolised and the enzymes responsible. Indicate any possible toxic metabolites which may be formed.

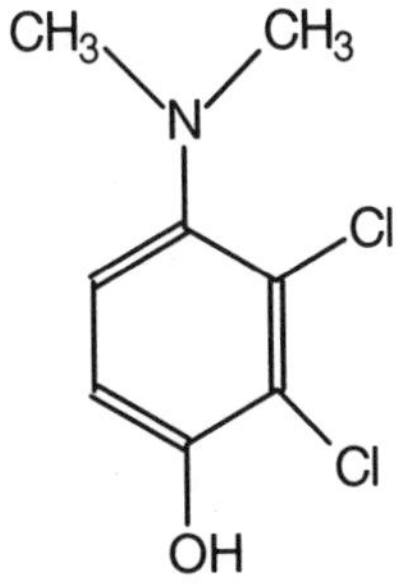

Figure: Question 16.

Q17. The chemical structure shown below is a potential fungicide being developed by a company. Toxicologists in the safety evaluation department need to know the likely metabolic fate of the compound before carrying out ecotoxicological studies. Predict the metabolism of the compound, indicating the enzymes involved and the site of metabolism. For each of your metabolites suggest whether the water solubility would be increased or decreased compared to the parent compound.

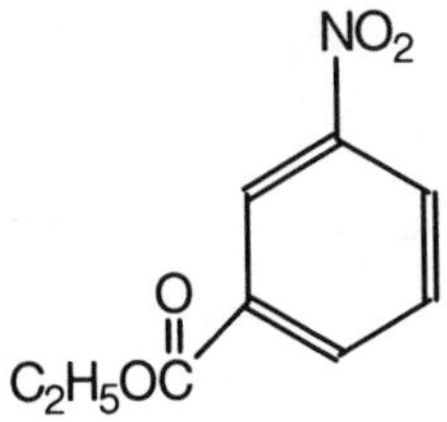

Figure: Question 17.

Q18. The structure shown below is a new chemical intermediate which is expected to be used in large quantities in an industrial environment.

(i)   Indicate what physicochemical data you would need to have for this compound in order to assess the likely hazard to the workforce exposed to it.

(ii)   Indicate the likely routes of metabolism.

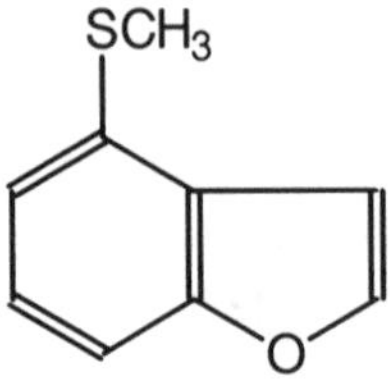

Figure: Question 18.

ANSWERS

MULTIPLE CHOICE

A1. (a) Man.

Man has the greatest size and surface area and of the species given will therefore have the slowest metabolic rate. Consequently the detoxication of the compound will be slowest and the toxicity likely to be the greatest.

A2. (d) Altered chemical structure.

Metabolism by definition involves alteration of the chemical structure of a drug. Although increased excretion and decreased toxicity may often also occur this does not always happen and increased toxicity may result.

A3. (c) Is a central part of the drug metabolising system.

Cytochrome P450 is the most important enzyme involved in drug metabolism. It is localised in the smooth endoplasmic reticulum and catalyses most of the phase 1 oxidation reactions.

A4. (d) The addition of an endogenous moiety.

Phase 2 metabolic transformations involve addition of a moiety derived endogenously which usually increases the polarity and water solubility. The moieties commonly involved are glucuronic acid, sulphate, glutathione and amino acids such as glycine.

A5. (b) A tripeptide.

Glutathione is composed of three amino acids: glutamic acid, cysteine and glycine (glutamyl-cysteinyl-glycine) abbreviated glu-cys-gly. It is involved in detoxication by conjugating with reactive metabolites, by reducing reactive metabolites and by reacting with and donating a hydrogen atom to free radicals.

A6. (a) True.

Cytochrome P450 catalyses phase 1 oxidation reactions.

A7. E.

All of these are involved in the operation of the microsomal enzyme system.

SHORT ANSWERS

A8. (a) Cytochrome P450 is a monooxygenase enzyme. It is found in many animal species in most tissues. The highest concentration is usually in the liver and it is located in the smooth endoplasmic reticulum. It exists in multiple forms (isoenzymes) which are grouped into thirteen families which form the P450 gene superfamily. /The enzyme is a haem-containing protein. It requires molecular oxygen and the coenzyme NADPH. It is associated with other enzymes such as cytochrome P450 reductase. It oxidises (and occasionally reduces) a wide variety of substrates, usually by adding one atom of oxygen, the other becoming incorporated into water.

(b) Glutathione is a tripeptide consisting of glutamic acid, cysteine and glycine (glu-cys-gly) and it has a free thiol (SH group). It is found in many tissues but is especially abundant in the liver where the concentration is about 5 mM. It reacts with and detoxifies reactive chemical intermediates (electrophiles) and free radicals. This detoxication may involve a chemical reaction or may be catalysed by glutathione-*S*-transferase enzymes.

(c) Phase 3 metabolism is the further metabolism of products of phase 2 metabolism. These are normally conjugates. For example, glutathione conjugates are further metabolised by removal of the glutamyl and glycinyl moieties. The remaining cysteine is then acetylated. The further metabolism of some cysteine conjugates by the enzyme CS lyase may produce toxic products. For example, the industrial chemical hexachlorobutadiene undergoes this route of metabolism and causes kidney toxicity as a result.

(d) The NIH shift is the term used to describe the chemical rearrangement which occurs during the cytochrome P450 mediated oxidation of aromatic compounds. The rearrangement was discovered at and reported by workers from the National Institutes of Health (NIH) in the U.S.A., hence the name. The phenomenon can best be illustrated in the oxidation of naphthalene (see figure page 51). When naphthalene is labelled with a deuterium atom at position 1, the products of cytochrome P450 mediated oxidation are 1- and 2-naphthols. In both products some deuterium is lost, but in the 1-naphthol product deuterium is found to have **moved** to the 2 position. In the 2-naphthol, some deuterium is replaced by hydrogen. This indicates that an epoxide intermediate is formed. The ratio of hydrogen to deuterium in the products and the ratio of 1-naphthol to 2-naphthol reflect the isotope effect of deuterium and are consistent with the postulated mechanism as shown in the figure below.

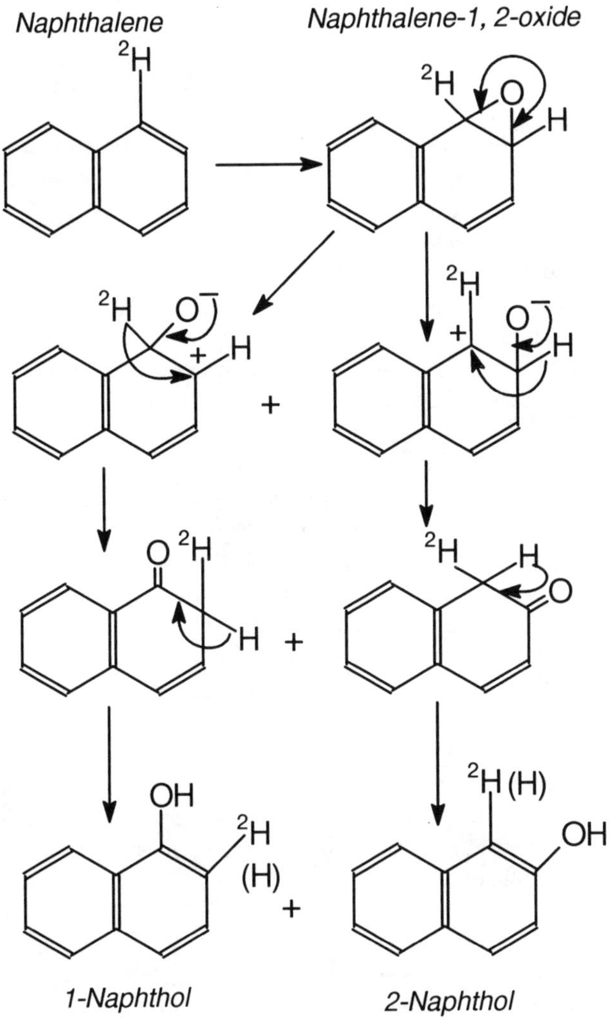

Figure: Answer 8.

A9. (a) Dealkylation is the removal of an alkyl (usually a methyl or ethyl group) from a molecule. The alkyl group may be attached to a nitrogen, sulphur or oxygen atom as indicated below. The dealkylation reaction is catalysed by the microsomal monooxygenase enzyme cytochrome P450 and involves an initial oxidation of the alkyl carbon atom followed by a rearrangement with loss of the oxidised alkyl group as an aldehyde (e.g. methanal or ethanal as indicated below). The other product is either an alcohol, thiol or amine as shown below:

$$R\text{-}O\text{-}C_2H_5 \quad\rightarrow\quad R\text{-}OH + CH_3CHO$$

$$R\text{-}NH\text{-}CH_3 \quad\rightarrow\quad R\text{-}NH_2 + HCHO$$

$$R\text{-}S\text{-}CH_3 \quad\rightarrow\quad R\text{-}SH + HCHO$$

(b) Alcohol dehydrogenase is an enzyme found in many animal species which catalyses the oxidation of alcohols to aldehydes. The coenzyme NADH is also required. There are several isoenzymes and a wide variety of alcohols are substrates. The enzyme is found particularly in the liver. There is evidence to suggest that there may be ethnic variations in the enzyme activity with Canadian Indians having reduced ability to metabolise ethanol.

(c) Glucuronic acid conjugation is the combination of certain foreign compounds with glucuronic acid to form glucuronides. Normally a carboxylic acid group or a hydroxyl group is conjugated to form ester or ether glucuronides. Occasionally thiol and NH glucuronides may be formed. The conjugates are water soluble and therefore readily excreted. The conjugation is catalysed by one of a group of glucuronosyltransferases. Glucuronic acid is a six carbon carbohydrate molecule formed from glucose-1-phosphate. For conjugation it is combined with uridine diphosphate (UDP) as UDP-glucuronic acid.

(d) Phase 1 metabolism refers to the first stage in the biotransformation of a foreign compound. The product will normally have a functional group added or an existing one modified which can be used as a "handle" for a second endogenous group, derived from intermediary metabolism, such as glucuronic acid to be added in phase 2 metabolism.

A10. (a) *N*-acetyltransferase is the enzyme which catalyses the acetylation of foreign compounds. This involves the addition of an acetyl group to a foreign compound. This addition is to an amine, hydrazine or sulphonamide group as shown below:

amine	R-NH$_2$	→	R-NHCOCH$_3$
hydrazine	R-NHNH$_2$	→	R-NHNHCOCH$_3$
sulphonamide	R-SO$_2$-NH$_2$	→	R-SO$_2$-NHCOCH$_3$

The donor is acetyl-CoA and there are two such enzymes in humans, NAT1 and NAT2. NAT2 shows a genetic polymorphism in humans which results in two phenotypes, rapid and slow acetylators. The enzymes are found mainly in cytosol and are widely distributed (e.g. liver, gastrointestinal tract, white blood cells).

(b) Epoxide hydrolase is the enzyme which catalyses the metabolism of epoxides in which water is added to the epoxide. The product is a dihydrodiol. The enzyme is found in the smooth endoplasmic reticulum in close proximity to cytochrome P450, especially around the centrilobular region of the liver, and it exists in multiple forms. Epoxide hydrolases have also been found in the cytosol and nuclear membrane.

(c) The glutathione-S-transferase is an enzyme which catalyses the addition of glutathione to foreign molecules. There are multiple forms of the enzyme (at least six) which are located in the cytosol but are also detectable in the endoplasmic reticulum. They are found in many tissues but particularly the liver, kidney, gut, testis and adrenal gland. The enzymes may accept a variety of different substrates but there is an absolute requirement for glutathione. The substrates do, however, contain an electrophilic carbon atom and tend to be hydrophobic.

(d) Taurine is a β-amino acid which is utilised in the conjugation of acids in some species, particularly the pigeon and ferret but also humans. The amino acid is synthesised from cysteine but is also absorbed from the diet. It is believed to have protective properties, especially in the heart and retina, and in the neutrophil it is believed to detoxify hypochlorous acid produced by myeloperoxidase. Cats, which utilise taurine for conjugation of bile acids, have an absolute requirement for dietary taurine and suffer retinal damage and cardiomyopathy if deficient in the amino acid.

PROBLEM SOLVING

A11. The metabolic pathways predicted and the enzymes catalysing them are shown in the figure (page 54).

(a) Cytochrome P450; (b) glucuronosyltransferase or sulphotransferase; (c) alcohol dehydrogenase; (d) aldehyde dehydrogenase; (e) epoxide hydrolase; (f) glutathione-S-transferase; (g) acyl CoA transferase and ligase or glucuronosyltransferase; (h) γ-glutamyltransferase; (i) glycinase; (j) acetyltransferase.

Figure: Answer 11. Possible routes of metabolism. GSH = glutathione; R = glucuronic acid or glycine; R₁ = glucuronic acid or sulphate.

A12. The phase 1 and phase 2 metabolic pathways predicted and the enzymes catalysing them are shown in the figure (page 56).

(a) Azoreductase; (b) amidase; (c) cytochrome P450; (d) glutathione-*S*-transferase; (e) γ-glutamyltransferase; (f) glycinase; (g) epoxide hydrolase; (h) *N*-acetyltransferase; (i) glucuronosyltransferase; (j) glucuronosyltransferase or sulphotransferase.

A13. The predicted metabolic pathways for this veterinary drug are shown in the figure (page 57). As the compound contains a nitro group, oral administration would be expected to result in reduction by the gut bacteria. This reduction would produce an aromatic amino compound which might be toxic to the red blood cells as are other aromatic amino compounds. Therefore an alternative route of administration would be preferable such as intravenous or subcutaneous injection.

(a) Nitroreductase; (b) *N*-acetyltransferase; (c) glutathione-*S*-transferase; (d) esterase; (e) alcohol dehydrogenase; (f) aldehyde dehydrogenase; (g) acyl CoA transferase; (h) ligase; (i) this fatty acid will be a substrate for the β-oxidation pathway; (j) cytochrome P450; (k) epoxide hydrolase; (l) glutathione-*S*-transferase; (m) γ-glutamyltransferase; (n) glycinase; (o) acetyltransferase.

A14. The predicted metabolic pathways for this veterinary drug are shown in the figure (page 58). As the compound contains a nitro group, oral administration would be expected to result in reduction by the gut bacteria. This reduction would produce an aromatic amino compound which might be toxic to the red blood cells, as are other aromatic amino compounds. Therefore an alternative route of administration would be preferable such as intravenous or subcutaneous injection.

(a) Nitroreductase; (b) *N*-acetyltransferase; (c) cytochrome P450; (d) glutathione-*S*-transferase; (e) epoxide hydrolase; (f) chemical rearrangement; (g) glucuronysyl-transferase or sulphotransferase; (h) γ-glutamyltransferase; (i) glycinase; (j) acetyltransferase.

Figure: Answer 12. Possible routes of metabolism. GSH = glutathione; G = glucuronic acid; R = glucuronic acid or sulphate.

Figure: Answer 13. Possible routes of metabolism. GSH = glutathione; R = glycine or glucuronic acid conjugates; R_1 = glucuronic acid or sulphate conjugates. # Dehydration may occur in the urine under acidic conditions. * Further metabolism of a glutathione conjugate is shown (pathways (m), (n), (o)).

Figure: Answer 14. Possible routes of metabolism. GSH = glutathione; R = glucuronic acid or sulphate conjugates.

A15. For the metabolic profile expected for the potential drug see figure (page 60). The amino group could be hydroxylated and this would produce first a hydroxylamine (reaction (h)), which is potentially toxic, and then a nitroso compound could result by chemical oxidation. Such compounds are known to be toxic to red cells.

(a) Cytochrome P450; (b) epoxide hydrolase; (c) glutathione-*S*-transferase; (d) γ-glutamyltransferase; (e) glycinase; (f) acetyltransferase; (g) *N*-acetyltransferase; (h) cytochrome P450; (i) glucuronosyltransferase; (j) dehydration in acidic conditions of urine may occur; (k) esterase; (l) glucuronosyltransferase or acyl CoA transferase and ligase; (m) alcohol dehydrogenase; (n) aldehyde dehydrogenase.

A16. The potential rodenticide would be predicted to be metabolised as shown in the figure (page 61). The demethylation of the substituted amine will produce a primary amine which can be hydroxylated and this could be potentially toxic. The aromatic ring may be oxidised via an epoxide which might be reactive and hence toxic. This is especially so given the presence of two halogen atoms.

(a) Cytochrome P450; (b) chemical rearrangement; (c) glutathione-*S*-transferase; (d) γ-glutamyltransferase; (e) glycinase; (f) acetyltransferase; (g) *N*-acetyltransferase; (h) glucuronosyltransferase or sulphotransferase; (i) epoxide hydrolase; (j) dehydration in the acidic conditions of urine may occur; (k) reversible (non-enzyme mediated) oxidation-reduction reactions may occur.

A17. The compound illustrated as a potential fungicide would be predicted to be metabolised as shown in the figure (page 62). The water solubility of metabolites resulting from pathways (a), (b), (c), (d), (g), (i), (j), (k) and (l) would be higher. The water solubility of the other metabolites would be similar to the parent compound.

(a) Esterase: this reaction would occur in many mammalian tissues including blood; (b) acyl CoA transferase and ligase: this would probably occur mainly in the liver; (c) glucuronosyltransferase: this would mainly occur in the liver; (d) nitroreductase: this would be most likely to occur in the gut bacteria; (e) *N*-acetyltransferase: this could occur in liver but also other tissues such as blood cells; (f) cytochrome P450: most likely and extensive in the liver but could occur in many tissues; (g) glutathione-*S*-transferase: most likely to occur in the liver as this is where the epoxide will be formed; (h) epoxide hydrolase: most likely to occur in the liver as this is where the epoxide will be formed; (i) γ-glutamyltransferase: this may occur in the kidney; (j) glycinase: this may occur in the kidney; (k) acetyltransferase: this may occur in the kidney; (l) sulphotransferase: this would probably take place in the liver where the hydroxylated metabolite is produced.

Figure: Answer 15. Possible routes of metabolism. GSH = glutathione; R = glucuronic acid; R_1 = glucuronic acid or glycine.

Figure: Answer 16. Possible routes of metabolism. *The glutathione conjugate will be further metabolised as shown (pathways (d), (e), (f), (j)). R = glucuronic acid or sulphate.

Figure: Answer 17. Possible routes of metabolism. GSH = glutathione; R = Glucuronic acid.
* Conjugation with sulphate is shown although conjugation with glucuronic acid, catalysed by glucuronosyltransferase, may also occur.

A18. (i) A knowledge of the volatility, boiling point, melting point and solubility in water and other solvents of this compound would be important. Also an indication of the chemical reactivity and stability would be useful. If the compound is a solid and would be used as such, the particle size might be important in terms of inhalation exposure.

(ii) The likely routes of metabolism are shown in the figure (page 64). The metabolic fate of the aromatic epoxide is as shown in previous examples (e.g. answer to question 7).

Figure: Answer 18. Possible routes of metabolism. GSH = glutathione; R = glucuronic acid. (a) Cytochrome P450; (b) glucuronosyltransferase; (c) glutathione-*S*-transferase; (d) γ-glutamyltransferase; (e) glycinase; (f) acetyltransferase; (g) epoxide hydrolase.

4

Factors affecting the toxicity of compounds

MULTIPLE CHOICE QUESTIONS

Choose one answer which you think is the most appropriate.

Q1. The acetylator phenotype is:

(a) not found in dogs
(b) found exclusively in Orientals
(c) responsible for the toxicity of amines
(d) an inherited trait affecting a particular metabolic reaction
(e) associated with the HLA type

Q2. The phenomenon of enzyme induction involves:

(a) an increase in the synthesis of the enzyme
(b) an increase in the activity of the enzyme
(c) an increase in liver weight
(d) a change in the substrate specificity of the enzyme
(e) an increase in bile flow

Q3. Piperonyl butoxide and phenobarbitone:

(a) are used in experimental studies to induce and inhibit the microsomal enzymes
(b) have no effect on drug metabolism
(c) uncouple electron transport in the mitochondria
(d) inhibit and induce the monooxygenase enzymes

Q4. Answer (a) if the statement is true and (b) if the statement is false.

The differences between species in susceptibility to the toxicity of chemicals are usually the result of differences in metabolism.

Question 5. Select A if 1, 2 and 3 are correct
Select B if 1 and 3 are correct
Select C if 2 and 4 are correct
Select D if only 4 is correct
Select E if all four are correct

Q5. The toxic effects of a chemical may be influenced by which of the following:

(1) kidney function
(2) body weight
(3) rate of metabolism of the compound
(4) time of day the chemical is administered

SHORT ANSWER QUESTIONS

Q6. Write short notes on the following using examples in relation to the toxicity of chemicals:

(a) hydroxylator status
(b) Clara cell
(c) teratogens
(d) disease

Q7. Write notes on/explain the toxicological importance of:

(a) cytochrome P450 2D6
(b) glucose-6-phosphate dehydrogenase deficiency
(c) protein deficiency
(d) chirality

Q8. Write notes on the role of three of the following in drug toxicity:

(a) ethnic origin
(b) cytochrome P450 isozymes
(c) enzyme induction
(d) acetylator phenotype

PROBLEM SOLVING QUESTIONS

Q9. The acute toxicity of a compound after intra-peritoneal injection was assessed in various species and the major organs examined for evidence of necrosis (+) or absence of necrosis (−):

Species	LD_{50} (mg kg^{-1} body wt)	Necrosis		
		Lung	Liver	Kidney
Rat (SpragueDawley)	23	+	−	−
Mouse (C57BL/6J)	23	+	−	+
Bird (Japanese quail)	75	−	+	−

Discuss these results and suggest possible explanations for the results obtained. Describe briefly further experiments you would carry out to test your proposals.

Q10. The compound shown below is a veterinary drug for use in a wide variety of animals including cats, dogs, pigs, birds and various types of monkeys. Show diagrammatically what routes of metabolism you might expect and point out any differences between the species.

Figure: Question 10.

$$CH_3CH_2OCCH_2 \qquad N=NCH_3$$

What factors might account for species differences in the metabolism and disposition of this compound?

Why is an understanding of species differences in metabolism important to toxicologists?

Q11. The acute toxicity of a compound was examined in rats. Control rats, rats pre-treated with phenobarbital (PB) and rats pre-treated with 3-methylcholanthrene (3MC) were given a range of doses of the compound. Any lethality was recorded and the pathological effects evaluated at post mortem.

		Necrosis		
Pre-treatment	LD$_{50}$ (mg kg^{-1})	Liver	Lung	Kidneys
None	75	+++	−	−
PB	23	+	+++	+
3MC	15	+	−	++++

Discuss these results and suggest possible explanations for them. Describe briefly any further experiments you would carry out to test your hypothesis.

Q12. Describe, with specific examples, how metabolism and factors which affect it may influence the toxicity of drugs in human patients.

Q13. Groups of five rats were pre-treated either with saline alone (control) or with phenobarbital (30 mg kg^{-1}) twice daily for 4 days or with benzo(a)pyrene (20 mg kg^{-1}) 24 hours before further treatment. The animals were then treated with the muscle relaxant zoxazolamine and the paralysis time and the plasma half-life ($t_{\frac{1}{2}}$) of zoxazolamine measured. The following results were obtained:

	Control	Phenobarbitone treated	Benzo(a)pyrene treated
Paralysis time (min)	137[a] ± 15	62[a] ± 21	20[a] ± 12
$t_{\frac{1}{2}}$(min)	102	38	12

[a] Mean ± standard error of the mean (SEM).

Explain these results and suggest experiments to test your proposals.

Q14. The following data were obtained in the safety evaluation of an industrial chemical (X) which was administered to rats daily in the diet for 1 month.

If the animals were pre-treated with hexachlorobiphenyl (i.p. injection) for 1 week before the exposure to the industrial chemical (X) started, the incidence of tumours was 50% after a daily dose of 2 mg kg^{-1}. Exposure to a single large dose of compound X (50 mg kg^{-1}) prior to the dosing schedule above reduced the tumours at all dose levels.

Dose of X (mg kg^{-1} day^{-1})	Incidence of liver tumours (%)
0	1
0.1	10
0.5	20
1.0	22
2.0	21

Discuss these results and suggest possible explanations for the data. What further experiments which you would carry out to prove your hypothesis?

Q15. The following data were obtained in a 90 day toxicity test in rats of a drug meant for repeated use by patients. How would you interpret these data and what other information from this study would be useful for this interpretation? What further studies would you propose in order to confirm your interpretation?

Dose (mg kg^{-1} day^{-1})	Organ weights (g) at post mortem (90 days)		
	Liver	Body	Thymus
0	10.2	352	0.40
10	12.1	310	0.34
20	14.5	250	0.22

Results are means from three rats.

Rats of equal starting weight were given the compound daily for 90 days administered in the food.

ANSWERS

MULTIPLE CHOICE

A1. (d) An inherited trait affecting a particular metabolic reaction.

The acetylation reaction in which the acetyl group (CH_3CO) is added to an amine, hydrazine or sulphonamide group is subject to genetic variation in humans. There are two phenotypes, rapid and slow acetylators which is a single gene trait governed by simple Mendelian inheritance with the rapid acetylator trait being dominant. This genetic trait results in a difference in the enzyme between the two phenotypes such that in the slow acetylators the enzyme, *N*-acetyltransferase (NAT2), catalyses the acetylation of substrates less efficiently than in the rapid acetylators. In the slow acetylators there are mutations in the gene coding for the enzyme, resulting in a relatively dysfunctional enzyme.

A2. (a) An increase in the synthesis of the enzyme.

Although the activity (and substrate specificity) of the enzyme may seem to be altered, in fact it is the synthesis of particular isozymes and their proportions which are altered. With some inducers liver weight and bile flow are increased, but not all inducers cause this.

A3. (d) Inhibit and induce the monooxygenase enzymes.

Piperonyl butoxide inhibits the monooxygenase enzymes, phenobarbitone induces this system.

A4. (a) True.

Species differences in toxicity are more commonly due to metabolic differences than intrinsic differences in sensitivity.

A5. E

All of the factors may affect toxicity. The kidney is the organ involved with excretion therefore a reduction in kidney function will tend to decrease excretion and therefore increase half-life and so increase the likely toxicity. The rate of metabolism may also influence toxicity by either increasing the production of a toxic metabolite or decreasing the removal of a toxic parent drug. Body weight may be a factor because unless the dose is adjusted an individual animal which is large will effectively receive less than a small one. Alternatively it may reflect the amount of body fat and this may sequester certain compounds thus reducing the acute toxicity. The time of day may influence the toxicity of a chemical if a part of the mechanism of toxicity involves a factor which shows diurnal variation. For example, glutathione levels in the liver vary throughout the day and hence if this is involved in detoxication dosing an animal at a time when levels are lower could increase susceptibility.

SHORT ANSWERS

A6. (a) Hydroxylator status is the term used to describe the ability of human subjects to carry out oxidation reactions, for example 4-hydroxylation of the drug debrisoquine. The ability to carry out this reaction has a genetic component. Hence individuals may be typed as poor or extensive hydroxylators. The variation resides in the enzyme cytochrome P450, the particular isozyme of which, 2D6, is deficient in some individuals (poor hydroxylators). Poor hydroxylators are more likely to suffer adverse effects of drugs as the blood/tissue level of the unchanged drug is higher in this group than in extensive hydroxylators.

(b) The Clara cell is one of the many cell types in the mammalian lung. It is metabolically active and hence may be a target for damage by certain chemicals. For example, the natural product ipomeanol is believed to be activated by cytochrome P450 in this cell type and subsequently damages it.

(c) Teratogens are agents (such as drugs or other chemicals) which cause defects or dysfunction in the developing embryo or foetus. Thus exposure of the female animal to teratogens during pregnancy may lead to malformations, growth retardation, functional deficiencies or death in utero. For example, thalidomide causes malformations in limbs leading to foreshortening. Alcohol may lead to low birth weight babies.

(d) Disease may be a factor which influences the toxicity of a chemical. Thus liver disease will tend to decrease the metabolism of some, although not all, drugs. By reducing the level of proteins such as plasma albumin, which is synthesised in the liver, liver disease may also affect the distribution of a drug and hence its toxicity. Similarly renal disease will alter the excretion of drugs and hence may increase toxicity. Disease may also affect the physiology and/or biochemistry of the body and therefore influence the metabolism or disposition of a drug in unexpected ways.

A7. (a) Cytochrome P450 2D6 is one of the isoenzymes of the cytochrome P450 system. It is responsible for catalysing the hydroxylation of debrisoquine and a number of other drugs. There are variations in the activity of this isoenzyme in the human population resulting from a mutation leading to an isoenzyme with reduced activity. Therefore individuals may be classified as extensive or poor metabolisers (hydroxylators) of debrisoquine. Poor metabolisers of debrisoquine have an exaggerated hypotensive effect after a therapeutic dose of the drug. With certain other drugs metabolised by this isozyme, poor metabolisers tend to have a greater susceptibility to certain adverse effects.

(b) The enzyme glucose-6-phosphate dehydrogenase is the first enzyme in the pentose phosphate shunt. Some human individuals have a genetically determined deficiency in this enzyme in the red blood cell. The genetic deficiency is sex linked, being only found in males with an especially high incidence in Sephardic Jews from Kurdistan. The enzyme is important as the reaction catalysed produces NADPH which is utilised in various pathways in intermediary metabolism. One of the toxicologically important uses of NADPH is the reduction of oxidised glutathione (GSSG) in the red blood cell. The maintenance of glutathione in the reduced (GSH) state is an important part of cellular protection. Thus GSH will reduce or remove, and thereby detoxify, reactive metabolites of xenobiotics. Those individuals who are deficient in glucose-6-phosphate dehydrogenase have low levels of reduced glutathione in their red blood cells that makes them especially susceptible to drugs which produce metabolites capable of oxidising haemoglobin in the red cell. Drugs such as primaquine and certain sulphonamides will thus cause haemolytic anaemia in susceptible individuals.

(c) Protein deficiency, occurring as a part of malnutrition, may result in the animal (human or other) showing either increased or decreased susceptibility to the toxicity of certain compounds. Protein deficiency will lead to a decrease in the level of glutathione as a result of a deficiency in sulphur amino acids such as cysteine. This will reduce the ability of the organism to remove and detoxify reactive metabolites and hence may increase the toxicity of some compounds. Protein deficiency will also result in a reduction in plasma proteins such as albumin, which will lead to reduced binding of some drugs and hence higher levels of free drug in the plasma. This may lead to increased toxicity. Reduced protein intake will also lead to a decrease in enzyme proteins such as cytochrome P450. This will decrease the ability of the organism to metabolise drugs and therefore may decrease toxicity if metabolic activation occurs. Alternatively if the parent compound is responsible for toxicity the decreased level of enzyme will increase toxicity.

(d) The presence of a chiral centre in a molecule results in isomers. Because biological systems involve receptors, proteins and other macromolecules with three-dimensional structures, different isomers may interact with such systems differently. Thus isomers may differ in the amount or the route of metabolism as a result of different affinities for a particular enzyme. Isomers may therefore have different disposition and different biological activity. Thus in some cases only one isomer may be active or toxic. Ability to separate isomers therefore may reduce the toxicity of a drug provided the active isomer is not also the toxic isomer. For example, the drug thalidomide exists as two isomers but one (S−) is more teratogenic than the other (R+).

A8. (a) The ethnic background of a human individual may be an important determinant of their response to drugs and other chemicals. This may be due to a difference in sensitivity/susceptibility or to a difference in disposition. Glucose-6-phosphate dehydrogenase deficiency increases susceptibility to certain drugs such as primaquine, resulting in haemolytic anaemia. This deficiency is found in male individuals of a particular ethnic origin, such as those who inhabit or derive from the eastern Mediterranean such as Sephardic Jews from Kurdistan. Altered disposition in particular ethnic groups often occurs as a result of differences in enzymes. For example, the acetylator phenotype is differently distributed in Orientals compared with Egyptians being mostly fast acetylators in the former but slow acetylators in the latter.

(b) The cytochrome P450 system, responsible for metabolising many drugs, consists of many isozymes. These have different substrate specificities and there is variation in the activity of these isozymes between species and individuals. Therefore absence of a particular isozyme in an individual or species might make them more susceptible to drug toxicity if the particular isozyme was responsible for a detoxication pathway. Conversely the individual or species might be less susceptible to a particular drug toxicity. The same also applies to susceptibility of a tissue to a particular drug toxicity, as isozymes vary in proportions between tissues within the same animal.

(c) The phenomenon of enzyme induction is the apparent increase in activity of an enzyme following the exposure of the animal to a xenobiotic. For example, repeated exposure to phenobarbital leads to an apparent increase in the activity of certain cytochrome P450 isozymes. This can be shown to occur with other enzymes involved with drug metabolism such as glucuronosyltransferase. The result is that the metabolism and therefore toxicity of a drug may be increased or decreased. This will depend on whether the drug or a metabolite is responsible for the toxic effect. For example, paracetamol toxicity to the liver is increased by induction of cytochrome P450 with phenobarbital in some species.

(d) Acetylator phenotype is a genetically determined characteristic in humans which determines the extent of acetylation of certain drugs. Isoniazid acetylation is affected by this phenotype. The phenotype is the result of a genetic difference between individuals resulting from mutations in the gene coding for

N-acetyltransferase 2. Thus slow acetylators have less functional enzyme than fast acetylators. The result is that detoxication by acetylation of hydrazines, sulphonamides and amines is decreased in slow acetylators. Toxic effects such as hydralazine-induced lupus and isoniazid-induced peripheral neuropathy are more common in the slow phenotype.

PROBLEM SOLVING

A9. The data shows that the two rodent species were similarly susceptible to the toxic compound in terms of LD_{50} and in each case the lung was one of the target organs affected. This suggests that the lung may be the target organ responsible for the lethality. Although damage to the kidney may prove fatal, this is less likely to be a cause of acute lethality than lung damage.

In the bird the toxicity in terms of lethality is much less (the LD_{50} is three times higher) and in this species the target organ is the liver. As with the kidney, liver damage is less likely to be the cause of acute lethality than lung damage. Thus the quail is less sensitive.

The reason for the species differences may lie in metabolic differences between birds and rodents. Thus the compound might undergo metabolic activation in the lungs of rodents but in the liver of birds. This could be due to differences in enzyme or isozyme complement in the different tissues. Alternatively the target organ difference may reflect a difference in distribution of either the parent compound or a metabolite in the different species. Thus in the rodent distribution and accumulation to the lung may be significant, perhaps because of a specific uptake system, whereas this may not be the case in the bird.

In order to test these hypotheses a number of experiments could be carried out. By using the radiolabelled compound differences in distribution could be determined between the species. This could be done using the technique of autoradiography for the whole animal or simply removal of the target organs and other tissues and determination of radioactivity by scintillation counting. This would also allow any covalent binding to tissues to be determined as an indicator of metabolic activation to potentially reactive metabolites. Following such *in vivo* studies, studies with the target organ tissue *in vitro* from each species could indicate if metabolic differences between these species are responsible for the target organ differences. This would involve using either crude tissue homogenates or subcellular fractions (e.g. microsomes) from the tissues. These studies would indicate if a tissue-specific difference was responsible or a combination of distribution and metabolism.

A10. Possible routes of metabolism for the veterinary drug are shown in the figure below (page 76).

(a) Azoreductase; (b) esterase; (c) acetyl CoA transferase and ligase; (d) alcohol dehydrogenase; (e) aldehyde dehydrogenase; (f) cytochrome P450; (g) epoxide hydrolase; (h) glutathione-*S*-transferase; (i) glucuronosyltransferase or sulphotransferase.

Factors which might account for differences in disposition:

(i)   As the compound, and more importantly, the metabolites resulting from bacterial action (pathway (a)) can be ionised, differences in the pH of the gastrointestinal tract may affect absorption by this route. Differences in skin type and thickness will affect dermal absorption.

(ii) Differences in breathing rate will affect absorption through the lungs.

(iii)   Differences in plasma proteins between species will affect binding of compounds to proteins and therefore distribution.

(iv) Metabolic differences will be influenced by diet and the presence/absence of particular enzymes. Thus dogs do not acetylate aromatic amines and cats and pigs do not utilise glucuronic acid and sulphate, respectively, due to enzymic differences. Availability of particular amino acids will influence preferred conjugation of the carboxylic acid in each species. Thus, some monkeys may utilise glutamine whereas birds conjugate with ornithine.

(v)   Different types of cytochrome P450 isozymes will be found in different species. This will influence whether a xenobiotic is metabolised and by what route. For example, in rats paracetamol is poorly metabolised via the toxic intermediate because of the relative lack of the cytochrome P450 isozyme responsible. Conversely, hamsters are very susceptible to the hepatotoxicity due to the presence of the particular isozyme responsible for the metabolism of paracetamol to the toxic intermediate.

An understanding of species differences in metabolism is vital for toxicologists as these differences often underlie the differences in toxicity seen between species and may help to explain them.

Figure: Answer 10. Possible routes of metabolism. # Glycine or glucuronic acid; R = glucuronic acid or sulphate. * Further metabolism is already illustrated on page 62.

A11. The compound administered to the rats was clearly toxic to several organs. In the control animals the liver was the main target organ for damage. However, this target organ shifted with pre-treatment of the animals. Although the liver was damaged to an extent in all cases, the lung and kidney also became targets.

The other data presented is the lethality. The LD_{50} is decreased in animals which have been pre-treated.

First, why might the liver be a target organ? If the compound is given orally then, after the gastrointestinal tract, the liver is the first major organ to be encountered. Also the liver is the metabolically most active organ and therefore may be a target even when other routes of administration are used.

Second, the fact that the target organ can be shifted by these particular pre-treatments of the animals suggests that metabolism is involved. Both phenobarbital and 3-methylcholanthrene are inducers of cytochrome P450 and therefore could be expected to change the metabolism of the compound if it is indeed metabolised. However, why should the target organ be shifted simply because of induction of cytochrome P450? This may be because particular isozyme levels are normally low in these organs and can be increased with a particular pre-treatment. The organs may also be targets because the disposition of the compound may result in the selective accumulation of the compound in these organs. The kidney would be exposed, however, as an organ of excretion.

The third point relates to the lethality. The fact that this increases with pre-treatment may be simply because of the target organ as damage to lungs and kidneys is more likely to be lethal than damage to liver (unless excessive). Alternatively, the pre-treatment may increase the production of a minor metabolite that is responsible for the lethal effect, which could be an effect on the central nervous system or heart rather than an effect on one of the organs indicated.

Further experiments should include a study of the disposition of this compound, perhaps using the radiolabelled substance. This should be carried out in control and pre-treated animals and should include a study of the binding of the compound to protein in the target organs. At the same time metabolic studies should be carried out to determine the metabolic profile and the effect on this of the pre-treatments. *In vitro* studies should include using homogenates and fractions from the three tissues from control and pre-treated animals to evaluate the metabolic capabilities of these tissues.

A12. The metabolism of a compound is a major determinant of the disposition and biological activity of many drugs. Therefore any factors which affect the metabolism of a drug will be most likely to affect its biological activity or the duration of that activity. The factors which may affect the metabolism of a drug in humans include genetic differences, the use of other drugs, exposure to other chemicals, disease, age, nutrition and sex.

The biological activity (either pharmacological or toxicological) of a drug may reside in the parent compound or a metabolite. If the pharmacological/toxicological activity resides in the parent compound then metabolism will decrease the activity. Factors which influence metabolism will therefore increase or decrease pharmacological or toxicological activity. Thus inhibition of metabolism by the administration of another drug or exposure to a food additive/constituent or environmental chemical may increase the pharmacological or toxicological effect. This will result in an increased half-life and an increased extent and duration of biological activity. For example, the genetically determined deficiency in the metabolism of drugs such as debrisoquine (poor metabolism or hydroxylation) leads to a higher plasma level of the drug after a therapeutic dose and therefore an exaggerated pharmacological effect (lowering of blood pressure). Conversely with the drug isoniazid those individuals who have a genetic predisposition to metabolise the drug more rapidly (rapid acetylators) have a reduced therapeutic effect (treatment of tuberculosis) compared with slow acetylators. However, the slow acetylators are more at risk from the hepatotoxicity and peripheral neuropathy that the drug may cause. The increased susceptibility to peripheral neuropathy is due to the higher plasma levels of the parent drug in the slow acetylator. The hepatic damage is due to inadequate detoxication of a reactive metabolite by acetylation. The hydrolysis of the muscle relaxant drug succinylcholine by esterases is also affected by a genetic deficiency leading to prolonged duration and exaggerated effect in those individuals who are deficient.

The interaction between two drugs is a common cause of toxic effects and may be a result of altered metabolism. For example, the antitubercular drug isoniazid inhibits the microsomal enzyme mediated metabolism of the anticonvulsant drug diphenylhydantoin. As the termination of the pharmacological effect of diphenylhydantoin requires metabolism, co-administration of isoniazid inhibits this and gives rise to increased half-life and problems of toxicity to the central nervous system. Similarly the antibiotic triacetyloleandomycin inhibits cytochrome P450 and when administered prior to drugs such as carbamazepine and theophylline may result in neurologic intoxication because of inhibited metabolism.

In contrast induction of enzymes of metabolism may influence toxicity. Thus use of the drug rifampicin, which induces cytochrome P450, increases the hepatotoxicity of isoniazid as a result of increased metabolic activation. In patients who have repeatedly used phenobarbital or alcohol, paracetamol overdose causes a more severe hepatic necrosis and dysfunction. This is as a result of induction of the metabolic activation of paracetamol.

The age of the patient, either old or young, may affect the metabolism of a drug and hence the duration and extent of its action. Thus young infants, especially those born prematurely, may be unable to adequately conjugate drugs with glucuronic acid. In the case of the drug chloramphenicol this may lead to cyanosis and death in such infants.

Disease, especially liver disease, may decrease the ability of the patient to metabolise the drug. For example, in patients with liver cirrhosis the half-lives of both chloramphenicol and isoniazid are prolonged due to decreased metabolism. Similarly malnutrition can result in decreased enzyme activity as a result of reduced protein intake and hence reduced protein synthesis. For example, reducing the protein intake of rats from 20% of the diet to 5% for 8 days results in a decrease in cytochrome P450 activity of more than 90%.

A13. The data shows that both the pharmacological effect and plasma half-life of zoxazolamine are influenced by the pre-treatments. Pre-treatment with phenobarbital leads to a decrease in the paralysis time and half-life and pre-treatment with the polycyclic hydrocarbon benzo(a)pyrene similarly leads to a much shorter half-life and greatly decreased paralysis time. The change in each parameter is of a similar magnitude after each pre-treatment.

The explanation is that the compounds used for the pre-treatments are both inducers of the cytochrome P450 enzyme system, that is they increase the activity of the enzyme system by increasing the amount of one or more of the isozymes which comprise the system. The drug zoxazolamine is metabolised by the cytochrome P450 system and consequently it is removed more rapidly in the induced animals. This is reflected in the plasma half-life, which decreases. As the muscle relaxation is due to the parent drug, the more rapidly it is removed by metabolism the shorter the duration of the pharmacological effect. The fact that the two inducers have a different quantitative effect on the duration of the effect and the half-life may be because the isozyme responsible for the metabolism of zoxazolamine is induced to a greater extent by benzo(a)pyrene than phenobarbital or that more than one isozyme is involved and the different inducers induce different proportions of isozymes. The zoxazolamine may indeed be metabolised more rapidly by the isozyme induced by benzo(a)pyrene.

In order to test these suggestions one could evaluate the metabolism of zoxazolamine in liver homogenates from animals treated with phenobarbital and animals treated with benzo(a)pyrene and compare the metabolites and rate of metabolism with liver homogenates from untreated animals. The metabolism *in vivo* could also be examined in pre-treated animals by measuring the metabolite(s) in blood and urine. An additional experiment would be to give animals an inhibitor of the cytochrome P450 enzyme system and measure plasma half-life and paralysis time of zoxazolamine. This should increase the half-life and paralysis time.

A14. The most striking aspect of this data is the unusual dose response for the tumour incidence. The maximum incidence is about 20% despite a fourfold increase in dose. The pre-treatment with hexachlorobiphenyl allows this to be increased to 50%. The tumours are induced by repeated daily exposure but giving a single large dose prior to the repeated exposure reduces the tumour incidence. All these factors point to saturation of some process. Saturable uptake might account for the low maximum tumour incidence but probably not the other observations. The most likely explanation is that metabolic activation is required to produce the tumorigenic agent and that the production of this reactive metabolite is saturable. The pre-treatment with hexachlorobiphenyl could increase the metabolism by inducing the required enzyme (e.g. cytochrome P450) and hence allow the animals to metabolise more of the compound and so increase the tumour incidence. Giving a large dose of the compound prior to repeated exposure might either saturate the enzyme for a period of time or irreversibly inhibit or destroy the enzyme and therefore the animal is unable to metabolise the compound to the tumorigenic agent.

These hypotheses could be tested by measuring the metabolism of the compound *in vivo* after various doses. This would indicate whether: a) metabolism occurred; b) whether it was saturable; c) whether exposure to a metabolite(s) correlated with the tumour incidence. The experiment could be repeated with animals pre-treated with hexachlorobiphenyl or a large dose of the compound to discover if the metabolism was increased and inhibited respectively. Finally the level and activity of likely enzymes could be measured in the liver (the target organ) after various doses to detect any inhibition or destruction of the enzyme.

A15. The data reveal that the compound causes an **increase** in liver weight and a **decrease** in thymus weight which appears dose dependent (although data for more doses is really needed to be certain of this). Also the body weight decreases with dose and therefore the increase in liver weight is not simply due to any increase in body weight. In fact this is more striking given the decrease in body weight.

The compound is therefore exerting toxic effects manifested as decreased body weight (a sensitive general indicator of an animal's state of health). The target organs would seem to be the liver and the thymus. Loss of thymus weight suggests atrophy or destruction of tissue. The increased liver weight could have a number of causes which further studies or information from this study could verify. The further information which should be available from this study includes: (a) food intake; (b) pathological evaluation of the liver and thymus. This information will indicate if the loss of body weight is due to a decrease in food, perhaps as a result of the presence of the compound in the food, or is due to another effect such as muscle wasting or altered intermediary metabolism. The pathological evaluation of the target organs will indicate if the thymus is undergoing atrophy or necrosis, loss of specific cell types or perhaps loss of fluid. Similarly the increase in liver weight may be due to accumulation of triglyceride (fatty liver), the presence of a tumour, hypertrophy or hyperplasia, proliferation of organelles (endoplasmic reticulum or peroxisomes) or the accumulation of fluid (hydropic degeneration). These can be determined by staining and light and electron microscopic examination and by biochemical (e.g. triglyceride or enzyme determinations) and other (wet weight/dry weight) techniques.

Depending on the results of these studies and the nature of the compound further studies using biochemical assays of target tissues might indicate whether microsomal or peroxisomal enzyme induction is occurring. Thus certain microsomal enzyme inducers such as TCDD (dioxin), which are responsible for receptor mediated induction, also cause thymic atrophy. Peroxisomal enzyme inducers may cause the appearance of liver tumours. Therefore the amount of cytochrome P450 and the activity of specific P450 isozymes and other enzymes such as catalase and palmitoyl CoA oxidase could be measured in microsomal and peroxisomal fractions. These data could confirm the hypothesis that the compound is a dioxin-like inducer of the microsomal enzymes, hence the increase in liver weight and the associated thymic atrophy.

5

Toxic responses

MULTIPLE CHOICE QUESTIONS

Choose one answer which you think is the most appropriate.

Q1. A chemical causes cancer in animals but is only positive in the Ames bacterial mutagenicity assay when S9 fraction is added. Is it:

(a) an ultimate carcinogen?
(b) a promoter?
(c) a proximate carcinogen?
(d) a non-genotoxic carcinogen?
(e) a co-carcinogen?

Q2. Chemicals which are active during the first week of pregnancy after fertilisation of the egg are most likely to cause which effect in the embryo:

(a) death
(b) malformations
(c) functional abnormalities
(d) growth retardation
(e) sterility

Q3. The drug thalidomide is a teratogen in humans. What is the major malformation it causes:

(a) aphakia
(b) phocomelia

(c) spina bifida
(d) anophthalmia
(e) cleft palate

Q4. The gestation period in humans is 9 months. What is the equivalent period in the rat:

(a) 12 weeks
(b) 21 days
(c) 45 days
(d) 15 days
(e) 15 weeks

Q5. Which of the following cause centrilobular necrosis in the liver due to a reactive metabolite:

(a) ethanol
(b) carbon tetrachloride
(c) bromobenzene
(d) paracetamol
(e) b, c and d

Q6. Carbon tetrachloride causes fatty liver mainly because of:

(a) increased uptake of fat from the diet
(b) increased secretion of fat from the liver
(c) increased mobilisation of fat from adipose tissue
(d) decreased secretion of fat from the liver
(e) decreased metabolism of fat in the liver

Q7. The hepatocytes in the centrilobular region of the liver:

(a) are less susceptible to hepatotoxic chemicals than other liver cells
(b) have a higher concentration of cytochrome P450 than other hepatocytes
(c) have a higher oxygen concentration than those in other regions
(d) have the highest glutathione content of any cells in the liver
(e) are located in zone 1

Q8. A teratogen causes defects usually because of:

(a) high exposure of the mother prior to fertilisation
(b) exposure of the female during organogenesis
(c) exposure of the male during spermatogenesis
(d) exposure of the neonate via the milk
(e) none of the above

Q9. Aplastic anaemia may be caused by:

(a) benzene exposure
(b) Fava beans
(c) treatment with methyldopa
(d) exposure to phenylhydrazine
(e) Primaquine

Q10. Heinz bodies are a manifestation of the toxic effects of a chemical on:

(a) lipids
(b) cytochrome P450
(c) haemoglobin
(d) the myelin sheath
(e) lymphocytes

Q11. Which of the following is not used for the detection of liver damage:

(a) plasma alanine transaminase
(b) urinary conjugated bilirubin
(c) alkaline phosphatase
(d) inulin clearance
(e) plasma albumin/globulin ratio

Q12. Which of the following is not used for the detection of mammalian kidney damage:

(a) urinary γ-glutamyltransferase
(b) blood urea nitrogen
(c) C-S lyase
(d) glycosuria
(e) α_2-microglobulin

Q13. In most species a depression in the level of the enzyme cholinesterase in the plasma indicates:

(a) liver damage
(b) myocardial damage
(c) organophosphate poisoning
(d) kidney damage
(e) none of the above

Q14. In a 90 day chronic toxicity study it was observed that both red and white blood cell counts were decreased. This is most probably the result of:

(a) an effect on the spleen
(b) an effect on the thymus
(c) direct toxicity to blood cells
(d) an effect on the bone marrow
(e) the induction of leukaemia

Questions 15, 16 and 17.   Select A if 1, 2 and 3 are correct
Select B if 1 and 3 are correct
Select C if 2 and 4 are correct
Select D if only 4 is correct
Select E if all four are correct

Q15. In drug-induced allergic reactions which of the following is true:

(1) there is no dose response
(2) only relatively large molecules are normally antigenic
(3) repeated exposure is necessary
(4) IgE is always involved

Q16. Adverse effects of drugs in humans may be caused by:

(1) exaggerated pharmacological effects after overdoses
(2) idiosyncratic effects after normal doses
(3) toxicity unconnected to pharmacological effect after inappropriate doses
(4) dietary constituents

Q17. One response to repeated exposure to chemicals is anaphylactic shock. This:

(1) results from the production of an antigen
(2) leads to a loss of blood pressure
(3) causes bronchoconstriction
(4) involves the immunoglobulin IgE

SHORT ANSWER QUESTIONS

Q18. Write notes on:

(a) ALT
(b) ototoxicity
(c) steatosis
(d) target organ toxicity

Q19. List the four types of immunotoxicity caused by chemicals. Give an example of a chemical which causes each type and a brief description.

Q20. Describe briefly the hapten hypothesis.

Q21. List the four manifestations of teratogenicity with a brief description of each.

PROBLEM SOLVING QUESTIONS

Q22. A new chemical is undergoing safety evaluation tests in rats. You have carried out some additional studies and the results are shown below. How do you interpret the data and what additional experiments would you suggest to verify your hypothesis?

Groups of rats	Dose X (mg kg^{-1})	Serum markers			Urinary markers	
		ALT	AST	Creatinine	Protein	γ-GT
Control	0	35 (20)	83 (21)	51 (3)	56 (4)	11 (3)
Control	100	444 (71)	1735 (97)	58 (7)	43 (2)	20 (5)
PB	100	4295 (244)	6479 (698)	52 (3)	35 (3)	14 (4)
Pip. butox.	100	248 (54)	703 (85)	101 (8)	161 (46)	131 (71)

Values are means (± SEM)
PB: pre-treated with phenobarbital, cytochrome P450 inducer.
Pip. butox.: pre-treated with piperonyl butoxide, cytochrome P450 inhibitor.
AST: aspartate transaminase.
ALT: alanine transaminase.
γ-GT: γ-glutamyltransferase.

Q23. A novel compound, X, is undergoing safety evaluation. It has to be tested for teratogenicity. Two doses are given to pregnant rats and the malformations present recorded at termination of pregnancy. The table below (page 89) shows the % malformations found after different exposure periods (days of gestation).

When administered to pregnant rats for the whole period of gestation compound X did not cause a significant increase in malformations at either dose (10 mg kg^{-1} or 30 mg kg^{-1}).

Interpret this data and suggest possible reasons for the results obtained. What further experiments do you think are necessary and what other information do you think is essential for a proper interpretation of the data?

Dose of X (mg kg^{-1})	Malformations			
	Days 7-9	Days 9-11	Days 11-13	Days 13-15
0	1%	2%	1%	1%
10	3%	12%	8%	5%
30	0%	1%	10%	7%

Q24. The following data were obtained in a safety evaluation study of a potential new drug. Pregnant female rats were exposed to the test compound given either as single doses on the day indicated or as three repeated doses covering the period of gestation indicated.

Single dose (10 mg kg^{-1})	Day 9	Day 10	Day 11	Day 12	Day 13
% Malformations	3	25	15	8	1
Repeated dosing (3 x 10 mg kg^{-1})	Days 8-10	Days 9-11	Days 10-12	Days 11-13	Days 12-14
% Malformations	1	8	10	2	0

Interpret and explain these data and suggest experiments which could substantiate your hypothesis. What other data should be available from the experiment described above and how might it help to explain the results?

ANSWERS

MULTIPLE CHOICE

A1. (c) Proximate carcinogen.

The compound requires metabolism by the S9 fraction which is the supernatant fraction of liver homogenate that remains after the homogenate is centrifuged at 9000 x g. This contains the microsomal enzymes (including cytochrome P450) which may be required for the metabolic activation. The compound is therefore not carcinogenic itself but requires an activation step.

A2. (a) Death.

Although teratogens may cause all of these effects, especially growth retardation during the first stage of pregnancy before implantation, organogenesis or functional maturation, the fertilised egg is more likely to suffer death following exposure to a chemical.

A3. (b) Phocomelia.

The major malformation observed after thalidomide was shortened limbs, termed phocomelia.

A4. (b) 21 days.

A5. (e) b, c and d.

All three compounds cause centrilobular hepatic necrosis, but alcohol only causes fatty liver and cirrhosis after chronic exposure.

A6. (d) Decreased secretion of fat from the liver.

Although carbon tetrachloride may affect various aspects of fat metabolism, the primary cause of fatty liver is inhibition of formation of the apolipoprotein involved in transport of triglycerides out of the liver. Hence secretion of lipids from the liver is decreased.

A7. (b) Have a higher concentration of cytochrome P450 than other hepatocytes.

Thus zone 3 or centrilobular hepatocytes have a higher concentration of cytochrome P450 than zone 1 or zone 2 hepatocytes.

A8. (b) Exposure of the female during organogenesis.

Classical teratogens such as thalidomide are active during the embryonic period when the limbs and other structural features are being formed, known as organogenesis. Although effects on the male and female gametes can theoretically cause birth defects this is less common.

A9. (a) Benzene exposure.

Aplastic anaemia is the loss of **all** blood cells as a result of damage to the bone marrow where the stem cells which are precursors to the blood cells are found. The other compounds cause other types of anaemia.

A10. (c) Haemoglobin.

Oxidative damage to haemoglobin in the red cell results in characteristic inclusion bodies in the red cell known as Heinz bodies.

A11. (d) Inulin clearance.

Inulin clearance is used for the determination of kidney function.

A12. (c) C-S lyase.

The enzyme C-S lyase or β-lyase is responsible for metabolising cysteine conjugates and is located in the kidney. It is not, however, used as a marker of kidney damage.

A13. (a) Liver damage.

If the level of the enzyme is decreased this is a result of liver damage as this is the site of synthesis. If the activity of the enzyme is decreased then this may be due to organophosphate poisoning in which the enzyme is irreversibly inhibited.

However, as normally measured it would not be possible to distinguish between these two effects.

A14. (d) An effect on the bone marrow.

The bone marrow contains stem cells which give rise to all the blood cells, therefore damage to this tissue leads to a decrease in both red and white cells.

A15. A.

All three parameters are characteristic of immunological (allergic) type reactions. However, the response varies, there being four basic types and there are several immunoglobulins which may be involved including IgE.

A16. E.

After overdoses or inappropriate doses of a drug the pharmacological effect may be exaggerated, for example excessive lowering of blood pressure. This is an adverse effect. Sometimes a drug may cause an adverse effect after therapeutic doses in particularly susceptible individuals. This is an idiosyncrasy. Inappropriate doses of a drug may cause unwanted effects not related to the expected/desired pharmacological effect of that drug. Occasionally there may be an interaction between a drug and a dietary constituent such as between monoamine oxidase inhibitor drugs and amines in foodstuffs such as cheese.

A17. E.

This immunological reaction involves all four of these factors.

SHORT ANSWERS

A18. (a) ALT is alanine transaminase (alanine aminotransferase; SGPT). This is an enzyme which catalyses the transamination reaction in which the amino group from alanine is α-ketogluterate. The enzyme is found in particularly high concentrations in the liver. During damage to the liver it leaks from damaged hepatocytes into the blood and may be detected there. When levels in the blood are elevated, liver damage is indicated. It therefore is used as a marker of liver damage although other organs may contain the enzyme and consequently other markers should also be measured.

(b) Ototoxicity is the term for damage to the ear, including any part of the auditory apparatus. Various chemicals affect the ear such as gentamycin and similar antibiotics, which damage the hair cells in the cochlear, and streptomycin, which damages the auditory nerve. Damage may be detected by histopathology and also by *in vivo* auditory tests using specific frequencies and electrophysiological measurements.

(c) Steatosis is the term for fatty accumulation in an organ. It is most commonly observed in the liver but may also be seen in the kidney and heart. It is usually due to the accumulation of triglycerides (normally) in the cells. This may be for various reasons: inhibited export due to inhibition of the synthesis of the apoprotein portion of the lipoprotein; increased uptake of fatty acids or lipids from the blood; increased synthesis of fatty acids; decreased breakdown of fatty acids; choline deficiency.

(d) Target organ toxicity is the specific damage to a particular organ in the body of an animal exposed to a chemical. This may occur because of a particular susceptibility of the organ to damage and inability to function after damage (e.g. heart), a particular metabolic pathway with which the compound interferes (e.g. liver), the ability of the organ to metabolise the compound to a toxic metabolite (e.g. liver), the facility of the organ to accumulate the compound (e.g. kidney), its position and blood supply (e.g. lung) or binding to a particular macromolecule (e.g. melanin in the eye).

A19. (a) Immunosuppression is the suppression of any part of the immune system, for example as caused by TCDD (dioxin) or tributyl tin.

(b) Immunostimulation is stimulation of the immune system, for example caused by synthetic cytokines.

(c) Allergy/hypersensitivity is the immune response to a foreign substance or a conjugate of a drug with a protein such as penicillin.

(d) Autoimmunity is an immune response initiated by a chemical in which the tissues of the body may be recognised as foreign and therefore attacked by the immune system. An example is the lupus erythematosus which is caused by the drug hydralazine.

A20. The hapten hypothesis explains the indirect immunotoxicological reactions which can occur in response to exposure to small molecules. In order for the immune system to recognise a molecule as foreign or non-self it needs to have a molecular weight greater than 3000-5000. However, small drug molecules with molecular weights smaller than this can still stimulate allergic reactions. This can occur if they are chemically reactive or are metabolised to chemically reactive metabolites which can then react with carrier proteins. The protein-drug conjugate is then potentially an antigen if recognised by the immune system as foreign. The drug or metabolite which is bound to the protein carrier is called a hapten.

A21. (a) Embryolethality involves the death of the embryo usually at an early stage such as before implantation. This leads to an abortion of the embryo.

(b) Malformations may result if exposure and damage/dysfunction to the embryo occurs during the organogenesis period when limbs and other structures are forming.

(c) Growth retardation may result if a teratogenic chemical reduces the rate overall of cell division at a very early or late (foetal) stage of gestation. This leads to a low birth weight baby or pup.

(d) Functional disturbances are the result of teratogenic chemicals generally affecting the later, foetal, stage of gestation when the organs such as the brain are developing functional rather than gross structural attributes.

PROBLEM SOLVING

A22. The compound causes elevations in the transaminases AST and ALT which suggest organ damage. The ratio of the two (approximately 1:3, ALT:AST) suggests that the liver is the target organ. Serum creatinine, urinary protein and γ-GT are not elevated and this suggests that kidney function is not compromised in the normal animals dosed with the compound. However, in animals pre-treated with phenobarbital, a microsomal enzyme inducing agent, toxicity as indicated by the serum transaminases is increased. This probably still reflects liver damage as the ratio is about 1:1.5, ALT:AST. No changes in serum creatinine or urinary parameters are observed. In animals pre-treated with the microsomal enzyme inhibitor piperonyl butoxide the rise in transaminases is much less although the ratio is still about 1:3, suggesting the liver is the target organ.

Thus, the effect of the pre-treatments suggests that the liver damage is altered by pre-treatments which affect the enzymes involved in the metabolism of foreign compounds. Increasing metabolism with phenobarbital increases toxicity whereas inhibiting metabolism with piperonyl butoxide decreases liver toxicity.

Overall this suggests a reactive metabolite is involved in liver toxicity. It can be observed that in the animals pre-treated with the enzyme inhibitor piperonyl butoxide, the serum creatinine and urinary parameters are also changed. Thus serum creatinine is significantly raised and protein and γ-GT in urine are also significantly raised. This suggests that although the liver toxicity of the compound is decreased by inhibiting the microsomal enzymes, kidney toxicity, as indicated by the urinary markers and serum creatinine, is increased. This could be due to: a) increased concentrations of the parent substance accumulating in the kidney as a result of blockade of the metabolism; b) another metabolite from an alternative metabolic pathway not blocked with piperonyl butoxide may be nephrotoxic; c) piperonyl butoxide may only block liver metabolism allowing more of the unchanged compound to reach and be metabolised in the kidney and cause damage.

If not available from the study described it would be important to verify by histopathology that liver and kidney damage have occurred as indicated by the data. In order to test these hypotheses it would be necessary first to evaluate the metabolism of the compound *in vivo* in control and pre-treated animals. This would indicate whether there was only one metabolic pathway or if there were more and what effect the pre-treatments had on this pathway(s).

Use of the radiolabelled compound would allow binding/accumulation of the parent compound and metabolites in the liver and kidney to be measured by autoradiography or direct measurement in excised tissue. The effect on this of the pre-treatments could also be evaluated. Other inducers and inhibitors of microsomal enzyme mediated metabolism might also be used to strengthen the hypothesis *in vivo*. Studies could be carried out *in vitro* in isolated liver and kidney tissue to determine the metabolism and susceptibility to the inhibitor of that metabolism in that specific tissue.

A23. Compound X is clearly teratogenic as it causes malformations at both dose levels and at a frequency clearly greater than in the control animals. The greatest percentage of malformations occurs after exposure during days 9-11 (10 mg kg^{-1}) or 11-13 (30 mg kg^{-1}), the periods during which organogenesis is occurring.

The fact that the higher dose causes fewer malformations at the early times than the lower dose could reflect embryolethality. Thus if the number of dead and resorbed early embryos is increased there will be fewer available to become malformed later. Therefore the fact that the maximum incidence of malformations is shifted towards a later time at the higher dose could be due to greater embryolethality at this dose allowing fewer malformations. In order to establish this the numbers of dead and resorbed embryos and foetuses need to be recorded as well as the number malformed.

When compound X was administered for the whole of the gestation period, no malformations were recorded. This again could be due either to a lethal effect on the very early embryo (fertilised egg or blastocyst stages) allowing few if any embryos to develop and hence no malformations. We do not know whether the number of dead and resorbed embryos was increased or how many normal embryos were produced in each case including control. This is necessary for a proper interpretation of the data. An alternative explanation is that the compound X has an effect on its own metabolism either in the maternal organism or the embryo. Thus if repeated exposure to the compound results in induction or inhibition of its own metabolism, then exposure to the teratogenic agent, whether the parent compound or a metabolite, might be reduced with this dosing regime.

Effects on the maternal organism may also be important and therefore any relevant observations should be recorded, including maternal body weight changes.

Additional data or experiments would include information about numbers of live, dead and resorbed embryos as well as malformed ones. Additional experiments to explain the data could include determination of the metabolism and disposition of compound X in the maternal and embryonic circulation after continuous dosing for the whole period and in 3 day stages. This might indicate whether induction or inhibition was taking place. Similarly comparison of metabolism and disposition after the two dose levels given at days 9-11 might indicate differences relevant to the difference in sensitivity. Such effects could also be investigated in maternal and embryonic tissue *in vitro*.

A24. The data show that the compound is teratogenic and that this is maximal on day 10 of gestation after a single dose with a significant percentage of malformations. This period of dosing is the period during which organogenesis is taking place in rats and is susceptible to interference. In the second experiment the same daily dose is given but is repeated for 3 days. The incidence of malformations is less. This could be due to the fact that repeated doses of the compound are leading to death of the embryo and abortion. The data presented do not indicate whether this occurs but this should be known from the experiment. Another explanation is that repeated dosing induces or inhibits metabolism of the compound so as to make it less teratogenic. This induction or inhibition may take place in the maternal organism or in the embryo itself. Induction of metabolism is more likely than inhibition.

Other data from the experiment will indicate whether the number of embryos is significantly less than in the control or between the treatments. This might indicate whether the apparent decrease in incidence of malformations is due to embryolethality. Signs of abortion and resorption may also be present.

Further experiments include measurement of the enzyme activity in embryonic and maternal tissue and metabolism of the drug *in vivo* after single and repeated dosing. This would indicate whether metabolism is increased after repeated dosing, whether alternative pathways are increased or whether metabolism is inhibited by repeated dosing and hence teratogenic metabolites are not produced. These effects could be due to induction of metabolising enzymes or inhibition of these enzymes. The latter could be due to reversible or irreversible inhibition or destruction of the enzyme.

6

Mechanisms of toxicity

MULTIPLE CHOICE QUESTIONS

Choose one answer which you think is the most appropriate.

Q1. Paracetamol is an analgesic drug which may cause liver damage after overdoses. This is the result of:

(a) depletion of body stores of sulphate
(b) inhibition of cytochrome P450
(c) production of a glutathione conjugate
(d) metabolic activation by the microsomal enzymes
(e) biliary excretion and metabolism by the gut bacteria

Q2. Indicate which of the following chemicals is metabolised to oxalic acid:

(a) methanol
(b) fluoroacetic acid
(c) ethylene glycol
(d) naphthalene
(e) benzene

Q3. Which of the following is the most important in determining the extent of toxicity of a chemical:

(a) chemical structure
(b) dose
(c) metabolism of the compound

(d) excretion of the compound
(e) metabolic detoxication of the compound

Q4. If an animal is exposed to the solvent benzene which of the following will be observed:

(a) benzene will be mainly excreted unchanged in the expired air
(b) benzene will be metabolised mainly to phenol and excreted as water soluble conjugated metabolites
(c) benzene will be entirely localised in body fat
(d) benzene will be excreted into the bile
(e) none of the above

Q5. Ethanol is used as an antidote for the treatment of ethylene glycol poisoning because it:

(a) facilitates the excretion of ethylene glycol
(b) blocks the metabolism of ethylene glycol
(c) increases the detoxication of ethylene glycol
(d) chelates ethylene glycol
(e) none of the above

Questions 6, 7 and 8.   Select A if 1, 2 and 3 are correct
                          Select B if 1 and 3 are correct
                          Select C if 2 and 4 are correct
                          Select D if only 4 is correct
                          Select E if all four are correct

Q6. In patients poisoned with aspirin the symptoms include:

(1) respiratory alkalosis
(2) metabolic alkalosis
(3) metabolic acidosis
(4) respiratory acidosis

Q7. Isoniazid toxicity to the peripheral nerves:

(1) is due to the parent drug
(2) only occurs in rapid acetylators
(3) is the result of depletion of pyridoxal
(4) is possibly due to a reactive metabolite

Q8. The hepatic toxicity of bromobenzene:

(1) is due to a glutathione conjugate
(2) is due to inhibition of cytochrome P450
(3) is decreased by phenobarbital pre-treatment
(4) is due to a reactive epoxide intermediate

PROBLEM SOLVING QUESTIONS

Q9. The plasma half-life of paracetamol in patients with liver damage due to overdosage is over twice that in normal human subjects after a therapeutic dose. Interpret this information in the light of what is known about paracetamol toxicity. Describe how data obtained in animal studies led to the formulation of an antidote.

Q10. Carbon monoxide is an important toxicant responsible for many deaths. Discuss briefly the mechanism of toxicity and describe how the poisoning is treated. Would a car mechanic exposed to 0.1% carbon monoxide in the air in a garage be at risk? (The concentration of oxygen in air is 21%; Haldane's constant is 240.) What factors might affect the extent of poisoning and the outcome?

Q11. The compound shown is a new herbicide designed to replace paraquat. Do you think it would show similar toxicity to paraquat? Explain the reasons for your decision in the light of the known mechanism of paraquat toxicity.

Figure: Question 11.

Q12. The following data in rats have been obtained for two hypothetical organophosphate insecticides.

Duration of toxicity (h)	Compound	LD_{50} (mg kg^{-1})	Time to onset of toxicity
48	Zapathion	12	30
6	Wimpathion	1300	120

In the light of the known mechanism of toxicity of organophosphate compounds, what toxic effects would you expect to observe after exposure to these compounds and what are the possible reasons for the differences between them?

How would you treat a victim poisoned with a compound such as Zapathion and what might occur if treatment was delayed?

Q13. The table below shows the effect of various combinations of treatments on potassium cyanide toxicity in mice. Interpret these data and explain the mechanisms underlying the effects of the treatments. Also, describe the mechanism of toxicity of cyanide.

	Treatment				
Expt no.	Hyperbaric oxygen	$NaNO_2$ $(g\ kg^{-1})$	$Na_2S_2O_3$ $(g\ kg^{-1})$	Dicobalt edetate $(mg\ kg^{-1})$	LD_{50} $(mg\ kg^{-1})$
1	$-$ [a]	0	0	0	11.8
2	$+$	0	0	0	11.2
3	$-$	0.1	0	0	21.2
4	$+$	0.1	0	0	21.3
5	$-$	0	1.0	0	34.8
6	$+$	0	1.0	0	39.0
7	$-$	0.1	1.0	0	51.7
8	$+$	0.1	1.0	0	73.0
9	$-$	0	0	15.0	94.0
10	$+$	0	0	15.0	93.0

[a] $-$ and $+$ indicate the absence and presence of hyperbaric oxygen respectively.

Mice were treated with sodium nitrite or sodium thiosulphate **before** being dosed with KCN or with dicobalt edetate, **after** being dosed with KCN.

ANSWERS

MULTIPLE CHOICE

A1. (d) Metabolic activation by the microsomal enzymes.

Although (a) and (c) are also true, metabolic activation to a reactive benzoquinoneimine, which interacts with tissue components, is the cause of the toxicity.

A2. (c) Ethylene glycol.

Ethylene glycol (often used in antifreeze) is metabolised via oxidation in several steps the first of which is catalysed by alcohol dehydrogenase, with the final end product being oxalic acid.

A3. (b) Dose.

Although all of the other factors may affect toxicity, the most important is the dose as toxicity is a relative phenomenon. Therefore at low enough doses there will be no toxic effect.

A4. (a) The benzene will be mainly excreted unchanged in the expired air.

As benzene is volatile it is readily expired through the lungs and this is an efficient and rapid process. It should be noted, however, that the benzene will also be metabolised to phenol and excreted as water soluble conjugated metabolites. The proportions being expired in the breath and metabolised and excreted in the urine as urinary metabolites will depend on the dose. Therefore at low doses a greater proportion will be excreted into the urine but as metabolism may be saturated at high doses more will be expired at such doses.

A5. (b) Blocks the metabolism of ethylene glycol.

The enzyme alcohol dehydrogenase metabolises both ethanol and ethylene glycol. Therefore there is competition between them. As ethylene glycol toxicity requires metabolism via alcohol dehydrogenase, the presence of ethanol, the preferred substrate, blocks this and so decreases the toxicity.

A6. B.

The symptoms of aspirin (or salicylate) poisoning include initial respiratory alkalosis which may proceed to metabolic acidosis.

A7. B.

The parent drug isoniazid is believed to react with endogenous substances similar to pyridoxal which leads to inhibition of formation of pyridoxal and hence a depletion of this coenzyme.

A8. D.

Bromobenzene causes hepatotoxicity via a reactive epoxide (2,4 epoxide) which interacts with tissue protein and other macromolecules in the liver, leading to necrosis.

PROBLEM SOLVING

A9. The plasma half-life of paracetamol is increased to twice the normal value after overdoses for several reasons. The liver is damaged by overdoses of paracetamol and hence its ability to metabolise paracetamol is compromised. This may be because of changes in intermediary metabolism, in blood flow and other physiological parameters. Secondly one of the major routes of metabolism of paracetamol is sulphate conjugation. Large doses of paracetamol deplete the body of sulphate and hence this route of metabolism is closed. The plasma level of unchanged paracetamol is therefore maintained at a high level. As the elimination of paracetamol is dependent on its metabolism, the half-life in the plasma becomes extended.

The other major pathway of metabolism, glucuronidation, may also become saturated even though glucuronic acid may not be limiting. The third pathway, formation of a mercapturic acid via glutathione conjugation, will also be compromised after an overdose, with depletion of glutathione. The reactive metabolite will therefore bind to hepatic protein, causing liver damage, or may be reduced back to paracetamol, so potentially increasing the half-life.

The initial animal studies with paracetamol revealed the following:

(a) Paracetamol was metabolised by cytochrome P450 to a reactive metabolite which bound covalently to liver protein as indicated with radiolabelled paracetamol.

This binding was located in the centrilobular area of the liver where damage was greatest.

(b) The tripeptide glutathione was depleted in the liver by large doses of paracetamol.

(c) The excretion of the mercapturic acid (*N*-acetylcysteine conjugate) of paracetamol was decreased by large doses of paracetamol in line with the decrease in glutathione.

(d) Depletion of glutathione with diethyl maleate increased the hepatotoxicity of paracetamol.

(e) The covalent binding and liver necrosis occurred at times and doses when glutathione levels had reached their minimum.

These findings indicated that glutathione was crucial in protecting the liver from damage. Therefore means were explored to replete glutathione in the liver. The most suitable solution proved to be *N*-acetylcysteine. Methionine will also increase glutathione levels but the synthesis from this source may be compromised by the paracetamol overdose itself.

A10. Carbon monoxide is a gas which is readily absorbed by inhalation. Once in the bloodstream, the molecule combines with the protein haemoglobin in the red cell, replacing oxygen and forming carboxyhaemglobin. This involves the molecule binding to the sixth ligand position of the iron atom at the active site of the haem molecule. Haemoglobin can bind four molecules of oxygen (or carbon monoxide). Fully saturated carboxyhaemoglobin therefore will carry no oxygen. The amount of oxygen carried will therefore depend on the degree of saturation. The binding of carbon monoxide is much tighter than that of oxygen and therefore will tend to dominate the haemoglobin. Also the bound carbon monoxide causes an allosteric change in the haemoglobin which distorts the oxyhaemoglobin dissociation curve such that any oxygen bound to the same haemoglobin molecule is released less readily. The result is that the oxygen dissociation curve is distorted as well as diminished and the ability of the vascular system to provide oxygen for the tissues is reduced much more than would be the case if carbon monoxide was simply equivalent to oxygen. Haldane described the reaction of oxygen and carbon monoxide with haemoglobin with an equation:

$$\frac{[COHb]}{[HbO_2]} = M \frac{[pCO]}{[pO_2]}$$

where M = Haldane's constant with a value of approximately 240.

Therefore to calculate the risk for the garage mechanic we use this equation. The partial pressure of the gases can be equated with the concentration. Therefore the values (given) are 0.1 for carbon monoxide and 21 for oxygen. Therefore the ratio of carboxyhaemoglobin to oxyhaemoglobin can be calculated:

$$\frac{[COHb]}{[HbO_2]} \; = \; 240 \text{ x } \frac{0.1}{21}$$

The ratio of COHb to HbO_2 is therefore 1.1, or more than 50% carboxyhaemoglobin. A concentration of carboxyhaemoglobin of 40-50% is around the threshold toxic lethal level. The concentration which could be achieved in the blood of the mechanic in this example with 0.1% carbon monoxide is therefore dangerous.

The risk would be greater if the mechanic was working only in a confined space with no source of fresh air or was not moving into a clean air environment. Also the person would be at more risk if they were breathing heavily such as during physical exertion. An individual with anaemia would be more at risk as the oxygen carrying capacity of the blood is already reduced.

A11. The compound would probably not show similar toxicity to paraquat for the following reasons:

(a) Paraquat has quaternary nitrogen atoms in a pyridine ring system (see figure). This arrangement allows the nitrogens to form free radicals which are able to be stabilised with the electrons from the double bonds in the ring. Hence the free radicals are stable. It is unlikely that the compound shown would be able to form stable free radicals as the rings are saturated.

Figure: Answer 11 (a). Structure of paraquat.

(b) The distance between the nitrogen atoms in paraquat is crucial for uptake into the cells of the target organ, the lung, via an active uptake system. This allows high concentrations to be achieved. In the compound shown this N−N distance is greater than in paraquat and therefore it may not fit the uptake system. Also the absence of charged nitrogens would probably preclude uptake as the natural substrates for the uptake system, polyamines such as putrescine, have two charged nitrogens, one at either end of the molecule.

Paraquat therefore is toxic to the lung by virtue of selective uptake via the polyamine uptake system which requires two charged nitrogen atoms 6.5 Å apart. This allows a high concentration to be achieved in the target cells. Furthermore the ability to accept electrons from donors such as NADPH and form a stable free radical is also important. The paraquat radical can donate its electron to oxygen, also present in high concentrations in the lung, and hence produce superoxide, which is toxic, via production of hydrogen peroxide and hydroxyl radical. This cyclical process involving the production of reactive oxygen species is called redox cycling.

A12. Organophosphate compounds cause toxic effects by binding to and inhibiting enzymes of the esterase type, especially acetylcholinesterase. This is because the structure has similarities to the natural substrate acetylcholine. Some organophosphates require metabolism before they will bind to acetylcholinesterase. It is not known with the compounds in the question whether that is required. The toxic effects of organophosphates are a direct result of the inhibition of the enzyme, resulting in an accumulation of the natural substrate, acetylcholine. The toxicity is therefore a result of accumulation of acetylcholine and the effects of excessive amounts interacting with different types of receptors.

Thus the effects expected can be defined by the type of receptor affected:

(a) Muscarinic effects: muscarinic receptors are found in smooth muscles, heart and exocrine glands. Symptoms of toxicity are tightness of the chest, wheezing due to bronchoconstriction, bradycardia and constriction of pupils (miosis). Salivation, lacrimation, sweating and increased peristalsis giving rise to nausea, vomiting and diarrhoea also occur.

(b) Nicotinic effects: nicotinic receptors are found in skeletal muscle and autonomic ganglia. Symptoms of toxicity are fatigue, involuntary twitching and muscular weakness which may affect respiration. Hypertension and hyperglycaemia may result from accumulation of acetylcholine at sympathetic ganglia.

(c) Effects on the central nervous system: effects on receptors in the central nervous system leads to the following symptoms of toxicity: tension, anxiety, ataxia, convulsions, coma, depression of respiratory and circulatory centres. The cause of death is usually respiratory failure due to neuromuscular paralysis, central depression and bronchoconstriction.

For the two hypothetical examples shown, the differences between them are in potency, speed of onset of toxicity (as indicated by lethality) and duration of effect.

Zapathion is markedly more toxic than Wimpathion. This could be for several reasons. For example, Zapathion may be a more potent inhibitor of acetylcholinesterase than Wimpathion. This may be due to the tightness of binding to the enzyme. Metabolism of Wimpathion to the active metabolite may be required first whereas this may not be the case for Zapathion or the extent of metabolism may be greater. Differences in distribution to vulnerable receptors due to differences in physicochemical properties could also be a factor.

The difference in the onset time could again be due to differences in metabolism: either the rate or routes of metabolism. There may even be no requirement for metabolism in the case of Zapathion, giving rise to more rapid effects. Alternatively the compounds may differ in physicochemical properties such as lipid solubility so that initial distribution may be very different. Thus if Wimpathion is very lipid soluble it will first distribute into body fat and only slowly redistribute to the tissues where the acetylcholinesterase and various receptors are located.

Differences in duration of action again may be for the same reasons. Thus a potent inhibitor of acetylcholinesterase will have prolonged duration of action whereas one which causes a more readily reversible inhibition of the enzyme will only be short acting. Rapid metabolism followed by excretion may remove the compound and therefore shorten the duration of action.

Treatment of a victim of poisoning with one of these compounds would involve primarily giving the antidotes pralidoxime and atropine. Pralidoxime displaces the organophosphate from the acetylcholinesterase and so regenerates the enzyme. Atropine antagonises the effects of excess acetylcholine.

If treatment with pralidoxime is delayed then the structure of the organophosphate-acetylcholinesterase complex may change or "age" and the enzyme is then irreversibly inhibited. This process often involves loss of an alkyl group attached to the phosphate group.

A13. The data show the effect of cyanide and various antidotes in mice. They reveal that a lethal dose of cyanide to mice is about 11 mg kg^{-1}. This is not affected by the use of hyperbaric oxygen but is reduced by the administration of sodium nitrite, cyanide being approximately half as toxic (LD_{50} higher). Again hyperbaric oxygen has no effect. However, with sodium thiosulphate the toxicity is reduced to about one third and hyperbaric oxygen may slightly reduce the toxicity still further (LD_{50} 34 vs 39). When both sodium nitrite and sodium thiosulphate are administered to mice, the decrease in lethality is greater than either but is approximately additive (LD_{50} 21 + 35 vs 52). Again, however, hyperbaric oxygen further decreases the toxicity. With dicobalt edetate as antidote the lethality is reduced to the greatest extent but hyperbaric oxygen has no effect.

It seems that hyperbaric oxygen increases the effectiveness of sodium thiosulphate either alone or combined with sodium nitrite. The mechanism underlying this is unknown and is difficult to explain as cyanide blocks the electron transport chain and thereby stops the utilisation of oxygen. Therefore oxygen should have no effect on the toxicity. The apparent effect must be related to the mechanism of action of sodium thiosulphate which helps to detoxify the cyanide by converting it, in a reaction mediated by rhodanese, to thiocyanate which is easily excreted in the urine.

The additive effect of sodium nitrite and sodium thiosulphate results from the fact that the antidotes operate in different ways. Sodium nitrite acts by converting haemoglobin to methaemoglobin which can readily bind cyanide to form cyanmethaemoglobin. The binding of cyanide to methaemoglobin is preferred over the binding to cytochrome oxidase in the mitochondrial electron transport chain. Therefore when methaemoglobin is present in the blood cyanide will bind to it in preference to cytochrome oxidase and hence mitochondrial function will be restored. However, cyanide still has to be eliminated and only a limited amount of methaemoglobin is tolerated by a mammalian organism. Sodium thiosulphate is given because it is required for the detoxication reaction catalysed by rhodanese which converts cyanide into thiocyanate, which is less toxic and is readily eliminated in the urine:

$$CN^- + S_2O_3^- = SCN^- + SO_3^-$$

Hyperbaric oxygen in some way may affect this reaction or the overall process.

Thus the two antidotes operate independently and therefore when used together their effect is additive.

Dicobalt edetate is the most effective antidote. This simply operates as a chelating agent, binding free cyanide in the blood, the whole complex being eliminated in the urine. Cyanide then diffuses away from the mitochondrial cytochrome oxidase as the concentration in the tissues falls.

The toxicity of cyanide is simply a result of a blockade of the electron transport chain which results in a deficiency of ATP and the inability to oxidise substrates such as succinate and NADH. Hence, cellular metabolism slows and tissues which cannot sustain an energy debt, such as the heart and central nervous system, fail. Death therefore is usually a result of cardiac failure.

7

Overall integration of the subject

PROBLEM SOLVING QUESTIONS

Q1. The compound shown below is a potential hypotensive drug. It may be given orally or via a skin patch and the parent compound is pharmacologically active. What routes of metabolism would you predict for this compound? Show these diagrammatically.

Would you anticipate that any genetic factors would affect the metabolism of this compound? If so would you expect such genetic factors to have any pharmacological or toxicological consequences?

Would you expect any differences in metabolism between the two possible routes of administration?

Figure: Question 1.

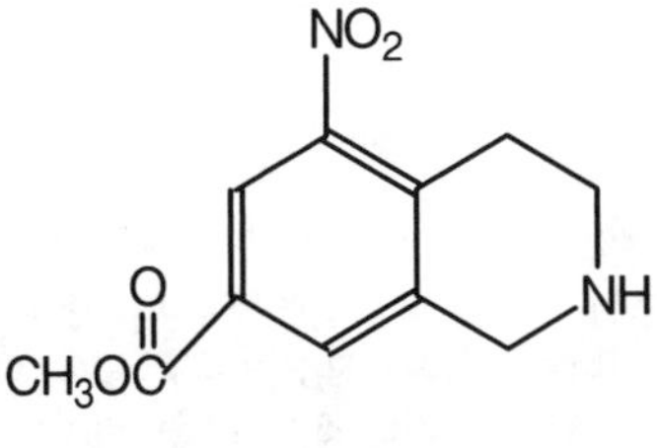

Q2. The data shown below has been derived from studies with a drug, X, in hepatocytes (cells from the liver) and adrenocortical cells (cells from adrenal gland). Each graph shows viability (measured as neutral red uptake) expressed as a percentage of control cells. In some cases cells have been treated with fructose, sodium fluoride or metyrapone. Fructose is a source of glycolytic ATP; sodium fluoride inhibits production of glycolytic ATP; metyrapone inhibits cytochrome P450.

How do you interpret this data? What additional experiments or controls would you suggest to support your conclusion?

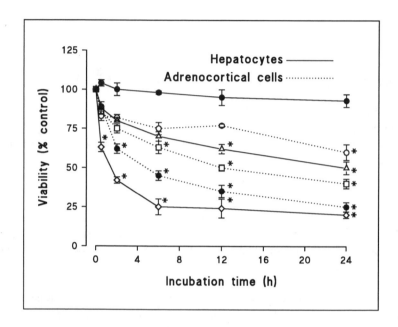

Figure: Question 2. Effect of drug X on viability (% control) in hepatocytes and adrenocortical cells. Hepatocytes: ●, exposed to 30 μM X; △, exposed to 30 μM X after sodium fluoride; ◇, exposed to 30 μM X after metyrapone. Adrenocortical cells: ●, exposed to 1 μM X; ○, exposed to 1 μM X after fructose; □, exposed to 1 μM X after fructose and sodium fluoride. Significantly different from control values, * $p < 0.05$.

Q3. The compound shown below (see figure page 113) has been designed as a new food colour. However, chronic exposure of mice to this compound administered in the drinking water resulted in a significant increase in incidence of lung tumours and other toxic effects (see table page 113). In rats, however, there was no such increased incidence of lung tumours. These effects were not observed at lower doses. The expected human intake would be 1 μg kg^{-1} day^{-1}.

From the structure of the compound, what likely metabolites would you predict from the data given and suggest possible mechanisms for the effects observed. What further experiments would you recommend in order to prove your hypothesis? From the data given would you advise the company to proceed with this compound as a food colour? Explain your reasoning.

Figure: Question 3. Compound designed as a food colour.

Species	Dose (mg kg^{-1} day^{-1})	Route of administration	Toxicity	Tumour incidence
Mouse	500	drinking water	red blood cell haemolysis	25%
Mouse	500	subcutaneous injection	none detected	19%
Mouse (control)	0	–	–	20%
Rat	500	drinking water	liver enlargement no haemolysis	12%
Rat (control)	0	–	–	13%

Q4. The data in graphs 1 (a)-(c) (page 114) were generated in isolated rat hepatocytes *in vitro*. The hepatocytes were exposed to various non-steroidal anti-inflammatory drugs (NSAIDS). Two (Ketoprofen and Flurbiprofen) are novel compounds which your company has synthesised. The data in graph 1(d) compares rat and human hepatocytes for Ketoprofen. The data in graph 2 (page 115) is from rat hepatocytes. Apart from Ketoprofen and Flurbiprofen all drugs are already in use in patients. Diclofenac and Piroxicam may cause liver damage, the others all cause gastric irritation and bleeding.

From the data which is the most toxic drug? Which of the two novel drugs would you advise developing? What other experiments do you think are necessary? What problems might result from the human use of Ketoprofen which were not detected in the *in vitro* system?

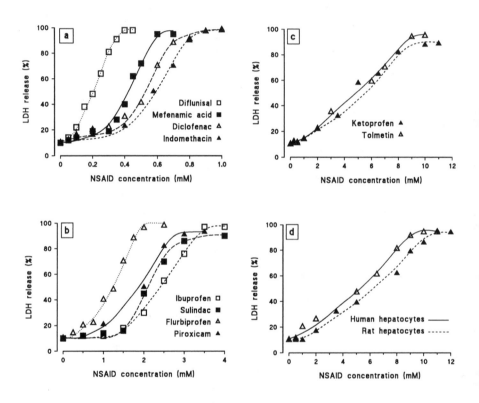

Figure: Question 4. Graphs 1 (a)-(d). (a)-(c): rat hepatocytes exposed to various non-steroidal anti-inflammatory drugs for 3 hours. (d): human and rat hepatocytes exposed to Ketoprofen for 3 hours. Cytotoxicity is indicated by leakage of lactate dehydrogenase (LDH), expressed as % total LDH in cells.

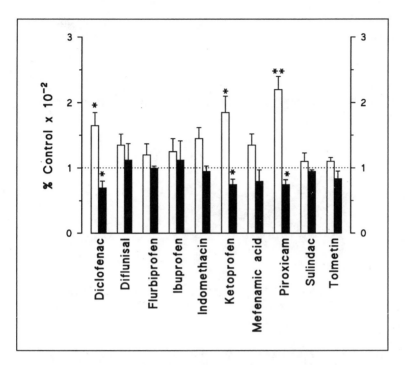

Figure: Question 4. Graph 2. Effects of pre-treatment of rats with phenobarbital (open bars) or SKF525A (shaded bars) on lactate dehydrogenase release from hepatocytes exposed to drugs for 3 hours. Data are expressed as a percentage of control. * $p < 0.05$ and ** $p < 0.01$ Significantly different from control. Phenobarbital and SKF525A induce and inhibit cytochrome P450 respectively.

Q5. The following data were obtained in a 28 day toxicity study in rats. The two compounds have been designed for combination therapy and repeated use in human patients.

Dose of A or B	Liver weight (g)	Body weight (g)	Thymus weight (g)
0	11.2	351	0.42
10 mg kg^{-1} A	10.4	337	0.30
1 mg kg^{-1} B	11.0	346	0.41
10 mg mg kg$^-$ A + 1 mg kg^{-1} B	14.3	325	0.26

Rats of approximately equal starting weight were given the compounds in food for 28 days. Results are means of 6 rats.

Interpret this data and devise a hypothesis to explain the results. What other information from this study would help your interpretation? What further experiments would you suggest which might help support your hypothesis?

Q6. The compound shown below is a potential pesticide intended for spraying onto edible crops.

Figure: Question 6.

Physical state = liquid; chloroform water partition coefficient (log P) = 3.2; b. pt = 40°C.

In the light of the information given:

(i) discuss the likely biotransformation in man;
(ii) comment on possible species variations in biotransformation;
(iii) comment on the expected absorption, distribution and excretion of this compound.

Q7. The following information on a potential new drug was gained at the termination of a two-year feeding study in rats. The drug was administered in the food. The drug is intended to be administered orally to humans on a daily basis for long periods of time, possibly a patient's lifetime.

Treatment	Body weight	Liver weight	Hepatic enzyme A	Hepatic enzyme B	Hepatic enzyme C
Control	650±50	14.9±1.4	3.9±0.5	30.2±2	1.4±0.2
Drug (1 mg kg^{-1} day^{-1})	520±37	35.8±3.5	216±38	38.0±4	1.9±0.1

Hepatic enzymes: A, carnitine acetyltransferase; B, catalase; C, ethoxycoumarin O-deethylase. All enzyme activities are expressed as nmol min^{-1} mg^{-1} protein. Values are means ± SEM of three determinations.

Discuss these data. In the light of your interpretation of the data and the expected pattern of use of the drug what other safety evaluation and metabolic studies would you recommend for this compound?

Q8. In safety evaluation studies of a new compound (SOP1) the following data were obtained when it was examined in rats and mice.

Species	SOP1 $(mg\ kg^{-1})$	Pre-treatment	Liver wt (% body wt)	ALT $(iu\ L^{-1})$	AST $(iu\ L^{-1})$
Rat	0	None	3.4	20	60
Rat	60	None	3.5	30	76
Rat	60	Pyrazole	4.6	500	120
Mouse	0	None	2.5	30	80
Mouse	60	None	3.5	700	1560
Mouse	60	Pyrazole	2.6	200	850

Pre-treatment: pyrazole specifically inhibits alcohol dehydrogenase but also affects some forms of cytochrome P450.

AST, aspartate transaminase; ALT, alanine transaminase. These are enzymes detected in the serum.

Discuss these results and suggest possible explanations for the data. Describe further experiments which you could perform to test your proposals.

Q9. The structure shown is an industrial chemical with the following characteristics:

chloroform:water partition coefficient at (pH 7.4) = 1280; b. pt = 85°C; m. pt = 13°C. The compound is to be used as an additive to lubricants for machine tools such as lathes.

Figure: Question 9.

Comment on the likelihood of human exposure and the likely routes of absorption.

Suggest ways in which the compound might be metabolised and the possible toxicity of the metabolites.

Q10. Estragole is a food additive. It has been shown to be carcinogenic in mice at a dose of 511 mg kg^{-1}. Estragole is metabolised to 1-hydroxyestragole and then to an electrophilic conjugate which is believed to be the ultimate carcinogen.

The table below shows the amount of metabolite produced by rats and mice. In humans the intake in food is 1 μg kg^{-1} and 0.3% is converted to the 1-hydroxyestragole. Interpret the data given and give your estimation of whether estragole in food is a significant hazard to humans. Explain your reasoning. If you were a regulatory toxicologist what other information might you require and how might this alter your assessment?

Dose of estragole (mg kg^{-1})	1-Hydroxyestragole				
	Rat			Mouse	
	#% dose	nmol kg^{-1} day^{-1}		% dose	nmol kg^{-1} day^{-1}
0.05	1.3	4.5		1.3	4.5
5	3.0	1020		2.1	714
500	11.4	387,600		7.8	265,390

#% Dose: percentage of estragole dosage converted to 1-hydroxyestragole.

Q11. The following data (table page 119) have been obtained in a toxicity study of a new chemical compound (SOP2) to be used to reduce corrosion in water systems. Rats were exposed to the compound in the drinking water at various concentrations for 3 months. The metabolism was found to occur via two pathways and the rate was determined for each of these over a 24 h period.

Discuss these data and suggest a hypothesis to explain the findings. How would you test your hypothesis?

What are the implications of these data for the toxicity testing of compounds?

Concentration of SOP2 in drinking water (mg L^{-1})	Volume of water drunk (ml 24 h^{-1})	Amount of SOP2 metabolised (µg 24 h^{-1})		% of animals with tumours in liver
		Metabolic 1	pathway 2	
12.8	28	180	34	2
64	29	645	465	7
128	25	960	1002	12
640	26	4160	5810	22
1536	21	6451	12920	24
2560	15	7102	16128	18

ANSWERS

PROBLEM SOLVING

A1. After oral administration the drug could undergo reduction by bacterial nitroreductases in the gut (see figure below). This will yield an amino group. This could undergo acetylation by acetyltransferases in the blood and liver.

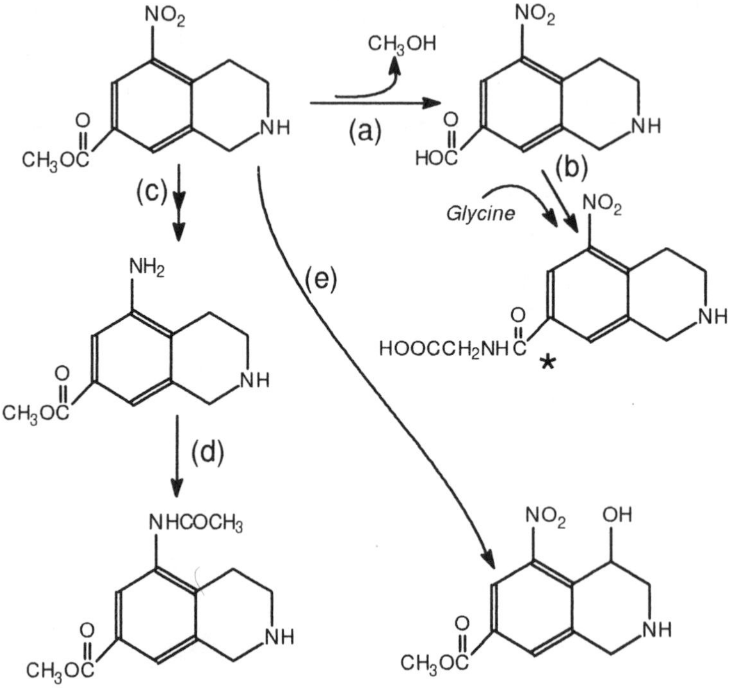

Figure: Answer 1. (a) Esterase; (b) acetyl CoA and ligase; (c) nitroreductase; (d) *N*-acetyltransferase; (e) cytochrome P450. * Conjugation with glucuronic acid may also occur in which case (b) is glucuronosyltransferase.

The ester side chain could be hydrolysed by esterases in the blood and other tissues to yield an acid. This could then be conjugated with an amino acid such as glycine or taurine or with glucuronic acid. The alicyclic ring could undergo hydroxylation. This may involve an isozyme of cytochrome P450 which shows genetic polymorphism. The structure of the compound is similar to the drug debrisoquine which is influenced by genetic variation in cytochrome P450 isozymes. Therefore the genetic factors which may affect this compound are the debrisoquine type of hydroxylation status and the acetylator phenotype. In the case of the hydroxylator status, this could affect the rate of removal of the parent drug. As this is the pharmacologically active compound there would then be a probable difference in dose response in relation to the effect of the drug between the two phenotypes. This would be an analogous situation to that with debrisoquine. However, the proportions and rates of the other routes of metabolism, hydrolysis and subsequent conjugation, reduction and subsequent acetylation would also be major factors in whether the genetic variations in cytochrome P450 did in fact increase the level of unchanged drug sufficiently to affect the pharmacological response to the drug. The acetylator phenotype would affect the removal and probable detoxication of the amino metabolite of the drug. Thus slow acetylators could be exposed to more of the reduced, substituted amino metabolite which might be toxic after further hydroxylation/oxidation.

If the drug was given via a skin patch then reduction of the nitro group would be unlikely. In this case acetylation also would not occur. Therefore the metabolism of the compound after administration via a skin patch could be more limited and more likely to be influenced by the genetic variations in cytochrome P450.

A2. The data show that drug X is not toxic to control hepatocytes but that the cytotoxicity is increased in the presence of sodium fluoride. This can be interpreted as suggesting that ATP is partially depleted by compound X and therefore when its reformation via glycolysis is blocked with fluoride, cytotoxicity occurs. The cytotoxicity of drug X is also increased by the presence of metyrapone, which is an inhibitor of cytochrome P450. This result suggests that metabolism of drug X by a cytochrome P450 mediated pathway is a detoxication process and so when inhibited toxicity occurs. In adrenocortical cells drug X is much more toxic than it is in hepatocytes (1 μM is more toxic in adrenocortical cells than 30μM in hepatocytes). However, the addition of fructose reduces the toxicity indicating that ATP depletion is involved in the toxicity of X. This is confirmed by the effect of fluoride in the fructose pre-treated cells in which toxicity of X is increased relative to the fructose treated cells. The toxicity of X may be greater to the adrenocortical cells for a number of reasons, such as increased sensitivity to ATP depletion or inadequate detoxication.

Further experiments could confirm such suggestions. Thus if inadequate detoxication is the reason for the increased sensitivity of the adrenocortical cells, this could be evaluated directly by measuring the metabolites of drug X in both cell types. A simpler experiment would be to treat the adrenocortical cells with the inhibitor metyrapone. This should have no effect if these cells are lacking in the detoxication pathway(s). Alternatively inducing cytochrome P450 in the adrenocortical cells by pre-treatment may decrease the cytotoxicity of X.

Additional useful information could include information about the cytotoxicity of drug X at different concentrations in the two cell types. The shift in the dose response curves due to the treatments could then be determined. This is preferable to measuring changes at one dose.

The reduced ability to tolerate ATP depletion could be investigated by giving a source of ATP, which should reduce the sensitivity of the adrenocortical cells. This has been done and although there is a small decrease, these cells do not become as resistant as hepatocytes.

In the experiments described there should also be control cells exposed to metyrapone, fructose and sodium fluoride alone.

A3. The compound seems to cause a small increase in the tumour incidence in mice exposed via the drinking water but not when given intraperitoneally. In the rat there is not really an increase in tumour incidence. However, the toxic effects are also different between the two species with the rat showing liver enlargement but no haemolysis whereas the mouse does show red cell haemolysis. However, the haemolysis only occurs when the compound is given to mice via the oral route. This suggests that the gut bacteria may be important. The structure contains a nitro group which can be reduced by bacterial nitroreductases in the gut ((a) in figure page 123). The resulting hydroxylamine metabolite may be responsible for the haemolysis. However, in the rat this may not occur. In the rat liver enlargement is observed, which could have a number of causes. Thus the production of tumours, the accumulation of fat or fluid, and the induction of microsomal or peroxisomal enzymes might all be reasons. The production of tumours and the accumulation of fat can be detected by histopathology, in the case of fat using specific staining with Oil Red O for example. The accumulation of fluid can be determined by measuring the wet weight of the liver and then the weight after drying in an oven. Induction of the microsomal or peroxisomal enzymes may be accompanied by an increase in the number of peroxisomes or amount of smooth endoplasmic reticulum. This can be observed by electron microscopy. It can also be determined quantitatively by measuring the activities of certain enzymes, by measuring the amount of enzyme protein or by measuring an increase in the mRNA specific for the induced enzymes.

The different effects in the two species could be the result of metabolic differences between them. This would have to be investigated by the analysis of urine and plasma for the metabolites of the compound. The role of the metabolites resulting from reduction of the compound in the toxicity could be investigated by using germ free animals (i.e. those without gut bacteria) or animals treated with antibiotics to remove the gut bacteria. The predicted metabolism is shown below (page 123).

Figure: Answer 3. Possible routes of metabolism. *Further metabolism of glutathione conjugates has been described in previous answers. (a) Nitroreductase; (b) azoreductase; (c) cytochrome P450; (d) *N*-acetyltransferase; (e) glutathione-*S*-transferase.

The products of reduction might be expected to be responsible for the haemolysis. The polychlorinated compound might be expected to be a microsomal enzyme inducer. Repeated exposure might therefore alter the metabolism of the compound and this should be investigated.

The doses of this compound given were high compared with the expected human dose and the metabolism may be different in humans especially at the intended daily exposure (the metabolism could be dose dependent).

The biochemical effects, metabolism and pathological effects should be determined at lower doses although the effects reported above were not observed at lower doses. The structure of the compound might suggest that the polychlorinated polycyclic hydrocarbon part of the structure could accumulate in animals exposed if this moiety is absorbed.

If the liver enlargement were due to peroxisomal proliferation then this is usually a rodent phenomenon. Many drugs and other compounds are microsomal enzyme inducers. However, this compound is proposed for use as a food colour rather than a drug. A knowledge of the mechanism underlying the toxic effects in both species would help a decision on whether to proceed. For example, if the production of tumours in mice could be linked to a particular metabolite this could be measured in human volunteers given a single dose of the food colour. Then a true dose ratio could be determined for comparison between mice or rats and humans and an informed decision taken. With this information the company could decide to proceed although the significant increase in tumours in one species may be sufficient to stop development.

A4. From the data presented (graph 1) it is clear that the most cytotoxic NSAID is Diflunisal based on leakage of the enzyme lactate dehydrogenase (LDH). Thus the approximate TD_{50} (concentration causing 50% LDH leakage) is 0.2 mM, which is a far lower concentration than any other drug.

From graphs 1 (b) and (c) it can be seen that Ketoprofen has a lower toxicity (higher TD_{50} which is approximately 5 mM) than Flurbiprofen (TD_{50} approximately 1.2 mM) *in vitro*. The dose response curve is also steeper for Flurbiprofen than Ketoprofen. Therefore it would probably be better to develop Ketoprofen. Even though the toxicity is increased (2x) by pre-treatment of animals with phenobarbital (graph 2) it is still less toxic than Flurbiprofen, the toxicity of which may also be slightly increased by phenobarbital pre-treatment. Also the rat and human hepatocytes show similar sensitivity for this drug, giving some indication that the *in vitro* data may be applicable to humans *in vivo*. However, there is no data on the therapeutic efficacy of the two drugs. Thus it may be that far higher doses of Ketoprofen than Flurbiprofen are required. It is therefore necessary to know the therapeutic index (TD_{50}/ED_{50}) in order to make a fully informed decision.

The fact that the cytotoxicity of Ketoprofen is significantly increased by phenobarbital and decreased by the inhibitor SKF525A should be investigated. The other two drugs for which this is important in this series are Piroxicam and Diclofenac, both of which may cause hepatic damage in humans. Therefore this might pose problems with Ketoprofen especially if patients are also being treated with drugs which induce cytochrome P450 or if patients have a significant intake of alcohol. Therefore animals which have been pre-treated with microsomal enzyme inducers should be dosed with Ketoprofen and evaluated for hepatic damage.

Although the hepatocyte is the target cell type in many instances involving metabolic activation, in some cases other organs may also be affected. Therefore serum clinical chemistry data should be scrutinised for indications of damage to other organs and histopathology should be carried out on other organs as well as the liver in animals in which the microsomal enzymes have been induced or inhibited. Thus induction may increase metabolic activation in various tissues including the liver and hence toxic effects may occur in those other tissues. Alternatively enzyme inhibition may block detoxication and lead to toxicity in other tissues. Knowledge of the metabolism of the two drugs would also be useful especially in relation to the other drugs which are known to cause hepatic toxicity.

Gastric toxicity or toxicity to other organs might arise with Ketoprofen which would not be detected in hepatocytes *in vitro*. Even though the rat and human hepatocytes were similar, other tissues in humans might be more susceptible.

A5. The compound A causes a slight drop in body weight and a pronounced drop in thymus weight. Compound B does not cause any such changes. However, the combination of A and B is more potent and causes a greater decrease in body weight and thymus weight than A alone. The combination also causes an increase in liver weight.

These data suggest that compound B is potentiating the effect of compound A which is toxic to the thymus. Compound B could be affecting the metabolism of compound A so that more of a toxic metabolite is being produced. The increase in liver weight is only observed with the combination of the two compounds. This again could be due to compound B changing the metabolism of compound A.

Further information obtainable from this study includes histopathology from the liver and thymus. This would allow any damage to be detected and assessed. The liver tissue could also be used for determination of the activities of microsomal monooxygenase enzymes and peroxisomal enzymes which may be induced by the treatments. Alternatively either compound may be an enzyme inhibitor. If B was either an enzyme inducer or inhibitor it might alter the metabolism of A in such a way as to increase its toxicity. Thus, a hypothesis which may explain the results is that compound A is metabolised by a detoxication pathway which is blocked by compound B. Compound B is not toxic to either the liver or thymus. The combination of A and B leads to either an increased level of unchanged A which is toxic to the thymus and causes increased liver weight or alters the metabolism of A so as to increase production of a toxic metabolite. The increased liver weight could be due to the enzyme induction caused by the parent compound or a metabolite which may be the metabolite responsible for the thymus toxicity. Similar effects are observed with TCDD (dioxin).

Further experiments would include evaluation of the metabolism of A and the effect on this of compound B. This would allow the hypothesis to be tested. The metabolites and parent compound could then be evaluated for their enzyme inducing properties and thymus toxicity.

A6. (i) The compound is likely to be metabolised as shown below (page 127) by the following pathways:

• reduction of the azo link by reductases especially those found in the gut bacteria (a): this will yield first a hydrazine compound, then a cleavage will yield methylamine and an aromatic amide.
• cleavage of the azide, hydrazide or amide link by esterases/amidases (c): this will yield 4-fluorobenzoic acid and either methylamine, methylhydrazine or azomethane.
• hydroxylation of the aromatic ring in the 2 or 3 position, mediated by cytochrome P450 and with an epoxide intermediate formed (e): the intermediate can then rearrange to a hydroxylated product, be hydrated by epoxide hydrolase to yield a dihydrodiol (h) or conjugated with glutathione (f).
• the glutathione conjugate so formed can then undergo further metabolism with loss of glutamyl (i) and glycinyl (j) residues to form a cysteine conjugate which will probably be acetylated (k) and under acidic conditions, such as in urine, lose water to form the unsaturated cysteine conjugate or mercapturic acid.
• the fluorobenzoic acid will be conjugated with glucuronic acid and/or an amino acid (d).
• the amide formed from azo reduction and cleavage could be acetylated (b).
• the ring hydroxylated metabolites(s) will be conjugated with glucuronic acid and sulphate (g).

In humans, which are omnivores, both glucuronic acid and amino acid conjugation will be utilised. The likely amino acids utilised will be glycine with possibly glutamine and taurine.

Figure: Answer 6. Possible routes of metabolism. R = glucuronic acid or sulphate. *Glycine or glucuronic acid. (a) Azoreductase; (b) N-acetyltransferase; (c) esterase; (d) acetyl CoA transferase and ligase; (e) and (l) cytochrome P450; (f) glutathione-S-transferase; (g) glucuronosyltransferase or sulphotransferase; (h) epoxide hydrolase; (i) γ-glutamyltransferase; (j) glycinase; (k) acetyltransferase.

(ii) As the compound is a potential pesticide, many species may be exposed. The most likely variation in metabolism between species will be the presence/numbers of gut flora capable of carrying out the reduction of the azo group (a). Then, as already indicated, there will be variation between herbivores and omnivores with regard to the conjugation of the 4-fluorobenzoic acid (d). Herbivores will tend to favour amino acid conjugation, carnivores glucuronic acid conjugation and omnivores a mixture of both. Similarly there will be variation in the conjugation of the ring hydroxylated metabolites (g) with some species utilising only sulphate conjugation (cats) and others (pigs) utilising only glucuronic acid conjugation and other species a mixture of both. If an amide metabolite is formed this could be acetylated. However, some species (i.e. dogs) do not carry out this reaction.

(iii) The physicochemical data given indicate that the compound is very lipid soluble (partition coefficient log P 3.2) and volatile (b. pt 40°C). Therefore it may be absorbed through the skin but will be very readily absorbed by inhalation through the lungs. The lipid solubility would probably mean that the compound would be distributed widely, especially into body fat. After inhalation, however, it would not be cleaved by reduction and therefore might be more persistent although it could still undergo hydrolysis. If hydrolysed to fluorobenzoic acid then this could be excreted into the urine without further conjugation as it probably would be ionised in aqueous media.

A7. The data show that the compound has a significant effect on a number of parameters. Body weight is decreased significantly in the treated group suggesting an adverse effect. However, as the chemical was administered in food the effect could be due to a reduction in palatability of the food and therefore a reduced food intake rather than a toxic effect of the chemical. Measurement of food intake would therefore be necessary to determine this.

The liver weight is markedly increased in the treated group. This degree of increase is unlikely to be due to microsomal enzyme induction or accumulation of fluid (lipid for example). However, it could be due to the presence of a tumour. As only one exposure level was used it is not known whether this increase in liver weight is dose related. The small increase in the activity of the liver enzyme C (ethoxycoumarin O-deethylase) suggests that microsomal enzyme induction may be occurring. However, the large increase in enzyme A and increase in enzyme B are consistent with induction of the peroxisomal enzymes in the liver. This induction would also be consistent with the large increase in liver weight. However, peroxisomal enzyme inducers may also be associated with the formation of liver tumours in rodents and therefore the increased liver weight could be due to a combination of increased numbers of peroxisomes and the presence of tumours. Therefore further information should be gained from the study carried out in rats to determine (a) if tumours are present and (b) to confirm that peroxisomal induction has occurred.

Further *in vivo* studies should be carried out in other species such as a non-human primate (the marmoset for example) in order to determine if the effects seen are specific to the rat. Metabolic studies should be carried out in the rat to determine (a) if the compound is metabolised and (b) if the metabolism is altered by repeat dosing. The structure of the compound and its metabolite(s) may suggest which is responsible for peroxisomal induction. Limited studies could be carried out in human volunteers to determine if the metabolic route in humans is the same as that in rats. However, studies could also be carried out in human hepatocytes and the results compared with those from rat hepatocytes. These studies could also include repeated exposure of human hepatocytes and determination of changes, if any, in peroxisomal number and enzyme content and activity.

As the compound is intended for repeated and long term exposure in humans, a knowledge of the effect of such exposure on the metabolism of the compound and on liver enzyme activities is essential. Provided that the human response and metabolism are different to those in the rat then the development of the drug could be continued.

A8. The compound SOP1 is clearly not toxic to the rat as there is no elevation of the transaminases or liver weight. In rats pre-treated with pyrazole, however, the compound causes significant elevations of the transaminases and liver weight is also increased. These data are consistent with toxicity to the liver.

In the mouse the compound is toxic, as indicated by the same markers, in normal animals whereas in pyrazole pre-treated mice toxicity is slightly decreased. Pyrazole inhibits alcohol dehydrogenase and some forms of cytochrome P450. Without knowing the structure it is not possible to speculate as to which enzyme is more likely to metabolise SOP1. The assumption is that the mechanism of toxicity is the same in rats and mice. Then if the parent compound is responsible for the toxicity, which would be consistent with the data in rats, the pyrazole is inhibiting the detoxication by either alcohol dehydrogenase or cytochrome P450. However, in the mice the converse is the case as toxicity is increased by pyrazole treatment. Therefore it is more likely that there is a toxic metabolite produced in both species which may be the same compound. In the rat the major pathway is catalysed by alcohol dehydrogenase or a pyrazole sensitive cytochrome P450 and another, minor pathway is catalysed by a different enzyme. The pyrazole sensitive pathway is a detoxication pathway and therefore when inhibited SOP1 is metabolised by a second pathway which leads to a toxic metabolite. In the mouse, the pathway catalysed by a pyrazole sensitive enzyme produces a toxic metabolite and so when inhibited (although not completely) the toxicity is decreased. This is shown in the diagram below (page 130).

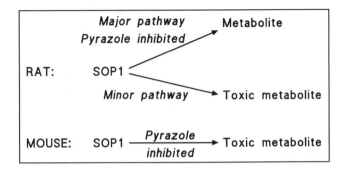

Figure: Answer 8.

There may be other pathways of metabolism for SOP1 in the mouse or other enzymes which produce the toxic metabolite but are not inhibited by pyrazole. It may be that the enzymes involved in the two species are similar but inhibited differently or that the enzymes are in fact different.

Further data needed includes the effect of pyrazole alone on the parameters measured (control data) and information about the structure of SOP1 and its metabolism in both species. With the basic metabolic information the effect of pyrazole and other inhibitors of alcohol dehydrogenase and inducers of cytochrome P450 on the metabolism could be evaluated. Knowledge of the identity of the metabolites would also allow these to be studied and so the hypothesis that a toxic metabolite is responsible could be tested directly. Thus rats and mice could be dosed with the metabolites and the toxicity determined.

A9. Although the compound shown may be a solid under some conditions, it is likely to be liquid at normal room temperature and is reasonably volatile (similar to methanol, for example, in terms of boiling point). It is very lipid soluble (log P is more than 3). The addition of this substance to lubricants for lathes means that workers will be likely to come into contact with the substance through their hands. Also the volatility of the compound means that it is likely, especially with working machines generating heat, that the vapour will be present around the machine. Consequently inhalation of the vapour is also fairly likely. Therefore the routes of absorption would be through the skin and via the lungs. The lipid solubility of the compound means that it would be well absorbed, especially through the lungs. Metabolism could involve oxidation, reduction and hydrolysis. Oxidation is most likely on the benzene ring (d) (see figure page 132).

Reduction is possible at the azo group (a). However, this would be more likely if the compound was ingested via the oral route and came into contact with gut bacteria.

Hydrolysis of the acetyl group might occur (a) to leave the azo compound or hydrazine if part reduction had taken place. Oxidation of the hydrazine group might also occur (d) and also oxidation of the methyl group.

The oxidation of the benzene ring will proceed via an epoxide and this may either be conjugated with glutathione (f), rearrange to a phenol or be hydrated to a diol (e).

The metabolite resulting from reduction might be toxic as the aromatic amino group could be oxidised to a hydroxylamine. Such compounds are known to cause haemolysis. Alternatively oxidation of the intermediate reduction product, the hydrazine or the parent compound on the azo group might produce toxic or carcinogenic metabolites (d).

The other potentially reactive metabolite is the epoxide (d). The presence of the fluorine atoms will increase the reactivity of this intermediate and it may react with glutathione and other thiols as does bromobenzene.

Figure: Answer 9. Conjugation with #*glucuronic acid or *sulphate. (a) Azoreductase; (b) esterase/amidase; (c) N-acetyltransferase; (d) cytochrome P450; (e) epoxide hydrolase; (f) glutathione-S-transferase; (g) γ-glutamyltransferase; (h) glycinase; (i) acetyltransferase.

A10. The data in the table show that in both rats and mice the proportion of the dose of estragole metabolised to 1-hydroxyestragole increases as the dose of estragole given is increased, i.e. the metabolism is dose dependent. Therefore at the high doses used the production of the metabolite is increased. In the human, the proportion metabolised is even less, being only 0.3% of the dose. Therefore with an intake of 1 μg kg^{-1}, the amount of 1-hydroxyestragole to which the human is exposed will be 3 x 10^{-3} μg kg^{-1}. The amount produced by mice at the carcinogenic dose will be 3.9 x 10^7 μg kg^{-1} (7.8% of 511 mg kg^{-1}). Therefore the dose ratio between the two species based on the metabolism is 1.3 x 10^{10}. In other words, the mouse produces 10,000 million times more proximate carcinogenic metabolite at the carcinogenic dose than humans do at the expected dose.

Furthermore estragole is carcinogenic in mice but not in rats therefore this may be a species specific response. Consequently the hazard to humans is very small. However, further information could help in determining the risk to humans. For example, as food additives are ingested repeatedly, is the metabolism of estragole altered by repeated exposure in humans? The compound could be an enzyme inducer or might be influenced by enzyme inducers and so more of the proximate metabolite could be produced. Is the metabolism dose-related in humans (this could be determined using human hepatocytes for example)? Does estragole produce tumours in other species and will the metabolite 1-hydroxyestragole produce tumours in all species or only in mice?

A11. The data show firstly that the drinking solution consumption by the rats decreases as the concentration of SOP1 increases. Could this be a reason for the decrease in tumour incidence? Closer examination of the data reveals that despite this decrease the amount of SOP1 metabolised by each pathway increases. Calculation of the amount of SOP1 consumed at each concentration level shows this increases. Calculation of the proportion of the dose metabolised by each pathway reveals, however, that 50% of the lowest dose is metabolised by pathway 1 but only 18% of the highest dose is metabolised by this route. In contrast, pathway 2 metabolises only 9% of the lowest dose but 42% of the highest dose. Therefore the major pathway switches from 1 to 2 at higher doses.

The data therefore suggest that saturation of metabolic pathway 1 may be taking place and pathway 2 then becomes more important. This may be the cause of the non-linearity in tumour incidence which reaches a maximum at only 24%. Thus the metabolite produced by pathway 1 may be responsible for the tumours. This hypothesis could be investigated as follows. If the metabolites are known from pathways 1 and 2 these could be administered to animals and the appearance of tumours monitored. The metabolism of SOP1 could be evaluated in vitro using liver homogenate from the same species of animal. The kinetics of the reaction would indicate whether saturation or substrate inhibition occurred in pathway 1.

The kinetic parameters for pathways 1 and 2 could be determined if the nature of the enzymes is known and can be isolated. Thus it is likely that the K_m of the enzyme for pathway 1 will be lower than the K_m of the enzyme for pathway 2.

The implications of this data are that knowledge of the dose response curve is essential as it may not be valid to extrapolate from high doses to low ones in situations where the dose response is compressed, as in this case. The toxic response, in this case percentage of animals with liver tumours, will therefore be higher than expected at low doses.